I0135238

Kama Sutra for Beginners

The Sex Positions Bible to Drastically and Rousingly Increase Libido with Your Partner. Discover Secret Tips and Tricks from Ancient Times...

© **Copyright 2019 by Eva Harmon - All rights reserved.**

The content contained within this book may not be reproduced, duplicated or transmitted without direct written permission from the author or the publisher. Under no circumstances will any blame or legal responsibility be held against the publisher, or author, for any damages, reparation, or monetary loss due to the information contained within this book. Either directly or indirectly.

Legal Notice:

This book is copyright protected. This book is only for personal use. You cannot amend, distribute, sell, use, quote or paraphrase any part, or the content within this book, without the consent of the author or publisher.

Disclaimer Notice:

Please note the information contained within this document is for educational and entertainment purposes only. All effort has been executed to present accurate, up to date, and reliable, complete information. No warranties of any kind are declared or implied. Readers acknowledge that the author is not engaging in the rendering of legal, financial, medical or professional advice. The content within this book has been derived from various sources. Please consult a licensed professional before attempting any techniques outlined in this book. By reading this document, the reader agrees that under no circumstances is the author responsible for any losses, direct or indirect, which are incurred as a result of the use of information contained within this document, including, but not limited to, — errors, omissions, or inaccuracies.

Table of Contents

Introduction

Congratulations on choosing this book and thank you for doing so! There are plenty of books on this subject on the market, thanks again for choosing this one! Every effort was made to ensure it is full of as much useful information as possible; please enjoy it! If you find this book useful in any way, a review on Amazon is always appreciated!

Disclaimer

Before we begin, there is one thing that I would like to mention. This book is not intended to replace medical advice. It is not responsible for the actions or the results of the reader. Please seek out the advice of a doctor before starting any health program. The author is not a medical doctor, and the information in this book is meant only to supplement your health decisions and actions, not dictate them. The wonders of autophagy are still being discovered as this book is being written. Please enjoy the information provided but also be wise in consuming it.

Introduction to the Book

The main focus of this book is to share strategies for maintaining a deep emotional connection with your long-term partner and how to accomplish this through the teachings of the Kama Sutra. Contained here are tips and suggestions on exactly how to continue to have an intimate and loving marriage for years and years from the perspective of the Kama Sutra.

What You Will Learn

In this book, we are going to delve into The Kama Sutra. This includes specific sex positions and techniques that you will learn about and can try with your partner in order to make your sex life more advanced than ever before.

I will begin by explaining what the Kama Sutra is, and I will share with you some ways that it can be incorporated into your own personal sex life. I will also share with you the other benefits of the Kama Sutra, such as how to increase intimacy, how to kiss and caress your partner, how to engage in rough sex and how a man can please a woman. After reading through this book, you will have a much deeper understanding of what the Kama Sutra can teach you about sex and love, and you will better understand the history of this guide.

Why This Information Cannot Be Found on Google

While there are many articles and blogs on Google that discuss the Kama Sutra, none of them are as accurate and as comprehensive as this book. Many online resources that focus on the Kama Sutra are only concerned with the sex positions, but there is so much more to learn and benefit from when studying this ancient text. In this book, you will find much more information than you would anywhere else. The Kama Sutra itself was not originally written in English, so this book is the best way to understand exactly what the teachings of the Kama Sutra entail.

As you will find out over the course of this book, the Kama Sutra is full of invaluable lessons that will change your sex life forever. Further, this book will not only improve your sex life but your relationship or marriage as a whole. The Kama Sutra is a book that contains deep and meaningful lessons about love, being in a relationship, sharing yourself with another person, different ways of demonstrating your love using physical touch, and much more. Through reading this book, you will find much more information than you would on the internet, as it breaks down the different sections of the Kama Sutra and presents them to you in a manner that is easy to digest, understand and implement in your own life. There is very little information on the internet regarding the Kama Sutra that goes as in-depth as this book does, and you will thank yourself for picking it up.

Chapter 1: What Is Kama Sutra?

We are going to begin this book by first learning a little bit about what exactly the Kama Sutra is. Then, we are going to learn a brief history of the Kama Sutra before we begin looking at how it can benefit you in the next chapter.

Firstly, what is Kama Sutra? When we say the term *Kama Sutra*, it is actually in reference to an ancient book. You may not have been aware of this fact, as most of the time we talk about Kama Sutra as a type of sex. While this book does guide you through sex by teaching you sex positions, it is actually a guide rather than a style of sex. Often, people will say "Kama Sutra Sex." As if it is a type of sex, when they are instead referring to a text. Throughout this book, you will see the term "The Kama Sutra," as I will be mentioning the book and its teachings.

You could say that the Kama Sutra is a guide to love and a guide to enjoying a pleasant life with your partner. This book can be seen as a guide to a long-lasting marriage that will help you to keep sex interesting. It will do this by showing you how to benefit from new forms of intimacy.

Common Misconceptions

Most often, the Kama Sutra is discussed in terms of wild and crazy experimental sex positions. There are numerous articles, blogs, and magazines that talk about the Kama Sutra in this way. The truth is, however, the Kama Sutra is a book that contains much more than just this.

You may have heard of Kama Sutra in conversations about sex or in articles that you read online. The truth is, however, this is a sacred book that was written long, long ago, which contains a guide for anyone who is looking to get more out of their relationship and their sex life.

A History of Kama Sutra

The book *The Kama Sutra* was written in Northern India. It was originally written in the language of *Sanskrit*. Sanskrit is an ancient Indian language. The original texts that gave rise to Buddhism were written in this language, which shows you just how much history is involved in the Kama Sutra. This book was written sometime around the second century AD, though nobody can be exactly certain of when.

The Kama Sutra is said to have been written by a man named *Vatsyayana*- who was an ancient Indian philosopher. It cannot be confirmed for sure if he wrote the entire book singlehandedly, but according to researchers, he made a significant contribution to the text.

The word *Kama* loosely translates to mean *affection, love,* and *desires*. This is quite telling, as the book is aimed at teaching the reader about all three of these factors. Affection, love, and desire are all very important when it comes to a long-term relationship or a marriage.

The Kama Sutra includes seven different sections or chapters. Each of these sections is focused on a different aspect of pleasure. These aspects of pleasure include both physical pleasure and emotional pleasure. Vatsyayana recognized that in a marriage, both forms of pleasure are equally important.

Only one of those seven sections contain sex positions, and the other six sections talk about a variety of other topics. These six sections each touch on a different category of sexual act or situation in which a couple can achieve a deeper level of intimacy. For example, kissing, touching, massaging, and so on.

Since the book was written in a time and place where it was surrounded by Hindu culture, it is considered disrespectful to the culture if the Kama Sutra is taken out of context. What this means is that it should not be read one single section at a time, rather it should be seen and consumed as a whole. This is because it was meant to be this way when it was written. The book is meant to be read all at once, from beginning to end. This allows a person to examine it in its entirety so that they can receive and benefit from the full scope of teachings that it contains.

What the Kama Sutra Contains

The Kama Sutra is a guidebook for love. Within the pages of this book are contained tips and tricks for everything involved in loving and caring for another person.

While the majority of times, the Kama Sutra is discussed in reference to the adventurousness of the sex positions it contains, this is only one small section of the book. The rest of the book contains a guide to many other forms of showing affection that does not include penetration. The Kama Sutra is said to be a guide to love, as it teaches its readers how to love and please their partner in a variety of ways.

The Kama Sutra was written with the intention that it would be read by men. This is likely because it was written so many years ago. The information that it contains pertains mostly to men who wish to attract and court a female partner. The book teaches men how to treat this woman whom he will eventually call his wife.

The Kama Sutra includes a guide to kissing, foreplay, loving touches, and other ways to achieve intimacy with your partner. These methods include bathing together and giving each other sensual massages- not necessarily the erotic kind.

The Kama Sutra also mentions same-sex relations in terms of one man having multiple women. It also touches on sexual encounters involving multiple men and one woman.

This book is full of information and tips for achieving a close emotional bond with your partner, which can be beneficial for any couple. As you can see, this book is much more than a book of wild sex positions.

When it comes to the section on sex positions, The Kama Sutra includes a variety of positions that range in difficulty level. It contains 64 sex positions in total. Later in this book, we will look at several of these sex positions in detail, including how to perform them and what benefits come of them. After reading about these sex positions and how to perform them, you can try to liven up your sex life by trying some of them out for yourself.

The Benefits

This book is full of information that can be useful in learning more about how to treat your partner lovingly in ways other than during sex. It can be useful whether or not you wish to learn more about sex positions in particular, as it can also help you to connect with your partner on a deeper level emotionally.

As your relationship progresses, it is important to keep sex and lust alive. When you become more and more comfortable with someone, the mystery and desire can begin to fade. This is completely normal. This happens because of the excitement of getting to know a person is no longer there. At the beginning of your relationship, everything you did together was brand new. At the beginning of a relationship, you are so eager to have sex with each other because the other person is new and hot and sort of like a novelty.

As you get used to being with your partner, it can be easy to lose those feelings of excitement and settle into the comfortability of your life together. This is by no means a bad thing. Getting to this point in your relationship is fun and comforting in its own way. This stage of a relationship is different from and in some ways, better than the early stages.

From a sexual perspective though, we don't want this stage of your relationship to bring with it the end of an exciting sex life. Introducing the concepts and lessons from the Kama Sutra can help you to maintain the lust and intimacy in your relationship. It can also provide you with new sexual adventures to take on together as an established couple.

The Kama Sutra contains a wealth of information about sex and different sex positions as well as including information about different positions from which to give massages, tips on kissing, and tips for men on courting women. There are a wide variety of sex positions included in this book, so there is no shortage of new positions to inspire you if you are feeling that your sex life is becoming stale. Information from this book can still be found to this day, even though it was written so long ago, not even in English!

The Criticisms

Though the Kama Sutra remains quite relevant to this day, several criticisms have been voiced regarding this ancient text and its contents, especially in recent years. In this section, we will examine three of the most popular criticisms that the Kama Sutra has received.

1. The Male Gaze

The Kama Sutra has received criticism for the way that it was written since it comes from the perspective of a man and discusses how to please a woman. Though this book mentions same-sex relations between two men, this is only in the context of men sharing one single woman. This can be seen as sexist to some.

2. Male Pleasure

Another criticism that has been voiced is concerning the way that this book discusses a man's ability to benefit from having many female sexual partners, and even mentions how he can have them all at one time. The Kama Sutra mentions that a man can have one wife and several mistresses, which is not a popular opinion in the year 2020.

3. Controversy

There has been debate about whether the Kama Sutra is a book that should be praised for the way that it teaches men how to prioritize intimacy and female pleasure, or whether it should be criticized for how it puts men in control in terms of sex. Even when it talks about relationships and love, it is written for a man who wishes to court his woman. Whichever way you view this book, it contains many valuable lessons. After reading this book, you are free to make your judgment about whether or not you think this book is still relevant.

4. Inclusion

Many people also think that the Kama Sutra should not be relevant anymore as it is not inclusive of different levels of ability and strength, as well as not including the potential for people with physical disabilities to try these positions.

5. Too Adventurous

For some, they may find that the Kama Sutra may seem like it is just a little too adventurous. Some people may think that this book full of positions that takes away from the deeper purposes of sex and simply wants to try to challenge the bodies of the couple during sex.

6. Realistic?

The Kama Sutra has been criticized for being a book that contains sex positions that are not realistic for the average human to try to recreate.

7. Sexism

This book has also been criticized for being sexist, as it is written for a man who wants to know how to please a woman physically and emotionally.

Chapter 2: Kama Sutra Tips and Tricks

Now that you have a solid understanding of what the Kama Sutra is and what it contains, we are going to go over some tips and tricks on how to get the most out of this book. After you read through this chapter, chapter three will focus on some of the specific techniques that the Kama Sutra contains and how you can begin to benefit from them.

What the Kama Sutra Can Do for Your Relationship and Sex Life

As I mentioned in the previous chapter, the Kama Sutra is not limited to the sex positions it contains. As you know by now, the Kama Sutra contains much more than this chapter alone. This is not to say that the chapter on sex positions is not of importance, as it can still provide you with a wealth of information about how to improve your sex life with your partner. For this reason, not only does the Kama Sutra give you tips and tricks for your relationship, but also some practical advice for trying new things in the bedroom.

How to Begin Talking About the Kama Sutra With Your Partner

It can be quite a difficult task, opening up to your partner about something that you wish to change about your sex life. This may be the first time you plan to have a serious conversation with them about sex. You may fear judgment or hurting their feelings, and you may fear that your partner will not be interested in what you are suggesting.

As we discussed in the previous chapter, your lust and desire for your partner may fade as time goes on. Using the information contained in the Kama Sutra can help you to keep your passion alive in the bedroom by providing you with new and exciting sexual adventures to embark on together.

You may feel unsure of how your partner will react to you telling them that you want to spice up your sex life. If you have been in this relationship for a while now and you feel that your sex life is becoming routine, chances are that your partner would agree with you. While this is true, your anxiety about bringing this up has likely increased the longer you have left this unsaid.

It is never a bad time to bring these topics up in conversation, regardless of how long you have been in the relationship or marriage. You deserve pleasure, passion, and lust, and sharing your thoughts with your partner should be a priority. Bringing up your desire for change can be seen as a conversation that will provide you both with benefits, rather than a critique. Letting your partner know that you are not criticizing them, but that you are simply looking for ways that you can both achieve more pleasure will show them that you mean no harm in bringing this up.

Begin by telling your partner that you have been reading about something called the Kama Sutra. They may have heard of this before, but it may help if you explain to them what the Kama Sutra is. As you know by now, many people have ideas about what the text is about, many of which are myths. Give your partner a background about the Kama Sutra, and tell them that you believe it can greatly benefit both of you in the bedroom.

Then, let your partner know that you have been interested in trying some of what you have learned in the bedroom with them. Explain to them what it is that you have wanted to try with them. Explain what it is and how it makes you feel. Whether or not you have tried it in the past with someone else, let them know that you would like to begin exploring it with them.

You can also ask them if there is anything that they have wanted to explore or talk about (that relates to sex) with you. This will open up a dialogue about sex and your sex life in general.

Finally, tell them that your goal is to improve your shared sex life and that you are open to any suggestions or conversations that they would like to share with you. Your sex dialogue should be a two-way street, so be prepared for a mutual exchange of thoughts and feelings.

Beginner Tips for Incorporating Concepts from the Kama Sutra in Your Life

The following subsection includes several tips for incorporating the Kama Sutra into your own sex life. This may be new for you, so follow the tips below to find out how you can get the most pleasure and benefit from this book.

Open Your Mind

Some of the concepts and sexual acts that you will learn about may be very new to you. While you do not have to do anything that you are uncomfortable with, try to read and understand with an open mind. These concepts may lead you to learn more about yourself and your partner.

Rediscover Your Partner

While you may know your partner like the back of your hand- especially if you have been together for some time now, it is important to remember that people grow and change. When it comes to incorporating new things in your sex life, your partner may surprise you with what they are open to and what they enjoy. As you begin to explore the Kama Sutra with your partner, try to view the experience as a rediscovering of each other. Rediscover their pleasure, their body, and their desires. Try to forget what you already know about them and view the experience as if you are learning about them for the first time all over again.

The beginning of any relationship comes with a lot of uncharted territories. You are exploring a new person's entire body- inside and out and letting them explore yours. This stage of discovery is something that we want to return to now and again during a long-term relationship or a marriage. This is because you should rediscover your partner's body as if it is the first time now and again.

People's desires change, and their bodies change. It is important to continue to learn and understand how best to please your partner as they grow and change. You should also expect the same from them in return. Revisiting your partner's body as if you know nothing about it can be a fun and flirty way to re-inject passion into your sex life. Try to remember the first time you had sex with your partner and channel that excitement and curiosity once again.

Trust Yourself

Trust yourself! At the most basic level, humans are animals. Just like any other animal, we are meant to have sex. This means that sex comes wired into our DNA and that we all have some knowledge of how to conduct ourselves during sexual intercourse. This is because our body can take over and follow its pleasure, its arousal, and its instincts. While you don't want to act like a complete animal in bed (unless you and your partner are into it), this is simply useful to keep in mind so that you can keep your nerves at bay. If you let your mind take control, it will get in the way of and inhibit this natural instinct that you came built with. Relaxation and being at ease will make the encounter much more enjoyable for both of you. If you are able to relax and enjoy the experience, your body will flow much smoother, and pleasure will come much easier to both you and your partner.

Communicate

It may seem like there is an expectation to pretend as you know exactly what you are doing and to seem like you have done it a thousand times before, but this is untrue. No matter who your partner is, they will be happy that you communicated and made sure that they were comfortable all along the way instead of pretending like you knew exactly what they wanted. Being able to communicate in bed is more impressive than not saying anything and guessing the entire time.

While some people may be embarrassed to be vocal and expressive in bed, many benefits can come of it, and many reasons why you may want to consider making a point to do this. By being vocal in the bedroom, you are able to communicate things to your partner without having to worry about ruining the mood or "killing the vibes." What this means is that you don't have to stop having sex or suddenly change your demeanor in order to talk to your partner during sex. By being vocal in the bedroom, you can communicate to them what you like, what you don't like, and what you want more of. This will make your enjoyment of sex better, and it will mean that you can experience more pleasure since your partner will know exactly what you want. You will also be able to please your partner better since you will know exactly what they want if they are vocal as well.

Express Yourself

Expressing yourself during sex allows you to express your pleasure. When you experience the physical bliss that is an orgasm, your body is always shocked at the level of pleasure it is feeling. If you have had an orgasm before, you know that the amount of pleasure you feel is so much that it begs to be let out in some way, usually by grasping something tightly or by screaming out in pleasure. By doing this, it actually enhances the feelings of your orgasm. Think of it this way- if you are experiencing an orgasm and you are holding your pleasure in so that you can remain quiet or because you are embarrassed about expressing yourself, your pleasure can only build to a certain level because there is no release for it. If instead, you let your pleasure out by exclaiming or grabbing onto the bed frame or a combination of the two, your pleasure can continue to build as it has an outlet. With no outlet, there must be a cap on it. Just like when you shake a bottle of soda, and it explodes out the top.

Expressing your pleasure during orgasm is very beneficial for your pleasure and for your sexual experience overall. At first, you may be unsure about how to do this, and you may be a little self-conscious about doing it with a partner. I can assure you, that your partner will most definitely be turned on by your exclamations of pleasure, as it will come as a sort of ego boost to them when they realize how much pleasure they caused you.

The first thing that you can do in order to become more comfortable with this idea is to try it on your own first. When it comes to anything sex-related, trying it first on your own is a great way to get comfortable with it before doing it with another person present. To try this on your own, do so when you are masturbating. This is a great time to try it as you are the person who best knows how to please yourself. Because of this, you can give yourself a strong enough orgasm- to the point where you will want to scream out in pleasure. When you come close to orgasm, open your mouth slightly. When you reach orgasm, allow whatever sounds escape your mouth to come out without holding them back and without judging yourself. You will likely find that you had an even better orgasm than usual because you weren't holding yourself back at all. You let your pleasure come about and let it out, which allows it to grow without putting a cap on it.

When you go to bed with your partner, try this same technique as you did when you were alone, and I guarantee that your partner will become extremely aroused by your orgasm sounds.

Understand Your Body and Your Mind

- The Body

The body is responsible for all of our physical sensations. The body houses all of our erogenous zones and our sexual centers. The body is our vehicle, and it is what allows us to feel pleasure at all. The body is responsible for our deep desires, our lust, our orgasms, our arousal, and our physical reactions to pleasure. There is something deep within that is not recognized by our conscious mind or our heart that moves us toward pleasure and away from pain. This is responsible for our deepest desires, and it wants desperately to seek them out.

The heart is the center of our body, and it provides us with our feelings of acceptance, warmth, comfort, happiness, and love. The heart is another important part of sex, and it is important for sexual comfort. If you are making love with someone whom you really care about, the heart will be where you feel those deep and intense feelings of inner warmth and connection.

- The Mind

The brain provides us with information about the situation we are in, allows us to use dirty talk, and makes our decisions, among other things. If the brain is distracted or tired or distressed, it will be very hard to know what we want, what we like, what we want to do, what to do next, etcetera. The brain is an important part of sex and sexual decision making.

Our emotions also play a large part when it comes to sex. While sometimes, we can perform the act of sex without emotions involved, this is not as sexually intelligent as we would like to be. Having sex with emotions does not mean that we are in love with every person we have sex with, but that we care for them, and we care for ourselves. It also means recognizing that we will have emotions surrounding desire, whether it is happiness, excitement, nervousness, joy. These emotions can all tell us something. Instead of blocking them out, we should be embracing them and listening to them. Being able to observe and read our own emotions, and the emotions of others is part of sexual intelligence. Emotions can also contribute to our enjoyment of sex as when we are feeling happy or in love. We tend to feel more intense pleasure when having sex with the person we feel strongly about.

The brain, the heart, and the body come together to form a sexual being, and this is responsible for all of our sexual preferences, desires, and comforts. It helps us seek out a partner and the activities that we get pleasure from. Being able to get in touch with your body means being able to look to all three of these parts of ourselves and listen to them as a whole and individually. This will ensure that you get the most out of your experiences with the Kama Sutra.

Chapter 3: How to Begin Practicing Kama Sutra

While you probably know how to please each other like it's second nature, rediscovering each other's bodies in a sexy way and learning new ways to please each other is great for couples who have been together for a long time. The Kama Sutra will help you to do this, and in this chapter, we are going to look at how you can benefit from this.

Where to Begin

Before beginning, we will first delve into the topic of the orgasm. We will look at the orgasm from both a male and a female perspective. We will look at the male body and the female body and how to please them, as well as how to give them a wonderful orgasm. This section will be helpful to you no matter how long you have been having sex, and no matter how long you have been with your partner.

Many people are out of touch with their sensuality, their desires, their fantasies, and even their bodies. By learning how to please the opposite sex, you will help your partner to discover their body and their body. This will also help you to become aware of this concerning your own body, and you will know how to get back in touch with all of these parts of your sexuality.

When it comes to sex, we all know that the cherry on top of a great session is the orgasm! There is no denying that an orgasm is the best part of being a creature that has sex for enjoyment and not solely to reproduce.

Understanding the Female Body

To give a woman an orgasm, you will need to understand the female body and all of the places that, when stimulated, will make a woman feel pleasure. Whether you are a female yourself or you are a male with a female partner, both sexes can benefit from learning more about the female body.

- The Clitoris

The clitoris is the place that many people know of as the spot to stimulate that is the easiest way to give a woman an orgasm. The clitoris is located very close to the vagina. It is a small bean-like structure that has many many nerve endings, which is why it can so easily lead to female pleasure. To find it, begin by placing a hand on the pelvic area, with the fingers towards the vagina. A woman can do this to herself, or a man can do this to find the woman's clitoris. Slowly move your hand downward, using your fingers to feel around. As you wrap your fingers underneath her, between her legs, feel around for a small lump-like structure. It is in a slightly different spot, covered by different amounts of layers and of different sizes on every woman, so explore around between the legs to find it. It will be towards the front of her body, right where her vaginal lips begin. On some women, you may even be able to see it with the eyes if there are not as many layers of vaginal lips covering it.

The clitoris is said to be the female penis. This is because it actually enlarges and becomes engorged when a woman is horny. It will be easier to find her clitoris if she is turned on. The clitoris is much larger than it seems, and this is because it extends up inside of the woman's body. Only a small part of it is located on the outside of the body, but the size of it is the reason why there are so many nerve endings located within and the reason why stimulating it will lead to such intense pleasure.

Once you have found the clitoris, you will then be able to stimulate it to give yourself or your woman an orgasm. Begin by gently placing two fingers on it and putting a bit of pressure. Rub it by moving your fingers in small circles- making sure to be gentle. Continue to do this, and she should begin to get more aroused the more you do this. By rubbing the clitoris, you will be able to stimulate the entire clitoris, even the part of it that you cannot see, and this will cause the woman to start to become wet in her vagina.

- The G-Spot

The G-Spot is a lesser-known spot than the clitoris, but a woman can have extreme amounts of pleasure if this spot is stimulated. To find this spot, you will need to insert a finger into her vagina. It is best to try to find this spot after you stimulated the clitoris for a bit because then her vagina will have begun to get wet- as it lubricates itself to prepare for penetration. You can use this to your advantage because it will make penetration more enjoyable for her and will reduce the friction of the entire vaginal area in general. When the vagina becomes very wet, it can lubricate the entire vaginal area, including the clitoris, which will then make it easier to stimulate the clitoris as well. No friction means smooth gliding, which results in pleasure and no pain. When she is wet enough, slide a finger inside of her vagina while she is lying on her back (a woman can do this for herself too) and make a "come here" motion with your finger, so that you are moving it towards her belly button. Feel around in this are, and when you feel a bumpy or rough surface, this is the G-Spot. Just like the clitoris, the G-Spot is slightly different for every woman, but they can all be in the same general area. The G-Spot will be a different size for different women, so be aware of this when trying to find it.

The reason that the G-Spot can give a woman intense pleasure is that it is actually connected to the clitoris. Inside the body, where the clitoris extends up into the woman, it meets the vagina, and this is the spot where the G-Spot is located. This thin wall between them allows for the pressure and stimulation to travel between them so that you are essentially also stimulating the clitoris when you are pleasuring her G-Spot.

To give a woman pleasure by stimulating her G-Spot, you will need to press on it over and over again until she reaches orgasm. This can be done using your fingers, your penis, or sex toys of a variety of sorts. We will talk about sex toys in a later chapter, but for now, we will look at the fingers and the penis. Stimulating this spot with your fingers is quite simple as you will have lots of control, and you will be able to feel around to see if you are in the right spot. When you have found the G-Spot with your fingers, gently press on it with the pads of your fingers and avoid curling your fingers around too much as you don't want your nails to scratch the inside of her vagina. Press with the pads of your fingers on her G-Spot with light pressure, but enough for her to feel what you are doing. Continue to do this, and you should feel her vagina getting increasingly wetter. As you do this, you can increase the speed of stimulation if she wishes. Communicate with her to see what she wants you to do (faster, slower, harder, lighter, deeper, shallower). A woman can do the same to herself in the bedroom. I just the same way, slide a finger inside of your vagina either with lube or after getting yourself a bit wet by watching porn or massaging your clitoris. Then, move your finger towards the front of your body and feel for the spot. Once you have found it, continue to stimulate it by putting pressure on it over and over again. It should feel good and get increasingly better the longer you do this. Eventually, the pleasure will build to a point where it feels as if you are about to orgasm. Continue to do whatever you were doing to get to this point, and orgasm will occur! This type of orgasm will be much more full body than a clitoral orgasm, as it includes the inside of the vagina and is also stimulating the clitoris from the inside.

The penis can also stimulate the G-Spot, but it is a little harder as there will not be as much control as there is when using fingers. Try to choose a position that will have the curve of the penis line up with the front of the vaginal wall, and this will give you the best chance of hitting the G-Spot. We will go into this further in chapter five, where we will look at specific positions. For now, though, knowing where the G-Spot is located as well as how to make a woman feel pleasure in that spot is a great start to being able to give her an amazing orgasm.

- The Anus

The anus is a very sensitive area for women, contrary to the beliefs of some people. While it is well-known that men have sensitive anuses and can receive pleasure here, it is a less well-known fact that so can women. Women have very sensitive anal openings because there are many nerve endings here and a lot of surface area. This means that when stimulated, a woman can feel a lot of pleasure here. Because this is an area that rarely receives stimulation. Therefore, when it does, it can be that much more enjoyable for a woman because she may not be used to the sensations.

The inside of the anus can give a woman lots of pleasure as well when stimulated. When a woman has her anus stimulated, it actually is only separated from the vagina by a thin layer, and similar to the clitoris and the G-Spot connection, she can actually orgasm from being anally stimulated because of the connection between her vagina and her anus. A woman can receive anal sex, and the penis making contact with her anal wall, especially the one toward the front of her body, can give her a very similar feeling to that of a vaginal orgasm.

The anus can also be stimulated with fingers, toys, or orally. Any of these ways can be enjoyable for the woman if she is open to receiving anal pleasure, as they will each give her a slightly different sensation. Think of how a warm tongue would feel vs. a smooth anal toy vs. the rough hands of the man she loves.

Understanding the Male Body

- The Penis

As we know, the male sex organ is the penis. A man can reach orgasm by having his penis rubbed, sucked on, kissed, or stimulated in a number of other ways. While you cannot easily tell when a woman is aroused, it is easy to tell when a man is aroused because his penis will become erect. This happens because then he can have sex with it- think of how hard it would be to have penetrative sex with a limp penis. When a man watches porn, sees a very attractive woman, or is touched in the right way, he will become erect. Then, by sliding his penis into a vagina repeatedly, into a sex toy like a fleshlight, or by having someone stroke it with their hand, he can eventually reach orgasm. Every man's penis is a different shape and a different size, and each man will like something slightly different in order to reach orgasm. There are so many things you can try and ways that a man could reach orgasm, there is lots of opportunity for exploration and trying new things.

We will revisit the topic of sex toys further in this book, so you will get more information on that very soon.

- The Testicles

A man's testicles may seem like they are there only to provide sperm for ejaculation, but they are also very sensitive erogenous zones for a man. If a man's testicles are stimulated, this can make him become very aroused and can make him erect if he wasn't already. A man's testicles can be stimulated during oral sex, during a handjob, or during sex in certain positions, and this will only add to the pleasure he is already feeling from having his penis stimulated in some way.

If you have ever had your testicles bumped in the wrong way, it definitely brought you a lot of pain for those few minutes afterward. Think of that level of pain but in terms of pleasure instead. This is what we want to unlock for you in your testicles. This level of sensation, but in the reverse- intense pleasure instead of intense pain.

Gently stroking the testicles with warm hands will get them used to touch so that they don't seize up and hug the body too closely. Gently rubbing the scrotum and massaging the testicles will add to whatever sexual activity is already happening. They can also be stimulated with the mouth during oral sex. The woman can move down to the testicles and gently suck or lick them to give a different sensation- that of warm moisture on sensitive skin.

A man can stimulate his own testicles while he is masturbating for added pleasure as well. If you are a man and you have never tried this, add it to your next masturbation session. Using one hand to stroke your penis and the other to massage your testicles will add a new dimension to your self-love sessions. Try this in the shower with a partner or without to enjoy the warmth or the water mixed with a massage and penis stimulation. You will never go back.

- The Anus

The anus is a well-known erogenous area of the male body. Males can get intense pleasure and even orgasm from being anally penetrated. This is due to the prostate gland being positioned right sat the spot where whatever is doing the stimulating would make contact with the anal wall. Right on the other side of this wall is the prostate, which happens to be extremely sensitive and leads to intense pleasure when stimulated in the right way.

A man's anus can be stimulated on the outside only, where-like a woman's, it is very sensitive due to a great number of very sensitive nerve endings being located there. This can be done using a tongue, fingers, a vibrating toy, or anything really. Beginning with this will lead the anus to relax and become receptive to being penetrated. Then, a sex toy or fingers can be inserted, and that's when the prostate will get its turn. When they prostate it pressed on over and over in a rhythmic pattern, it will cause a man to feel intense pleasure and eventually to reach orgasm. This is similar to the G-Spot in a woman where it needs to be continuously stimulated to eventually give her an orgasm.

Anal sex for a man is not just reserved for gay couples. Many heterosexual couples practice pegging, which is anal sex from a woman to a man using a sex toy. We will revisit this later, but this point is to say that the pleasure potential of a man's anus is not only reserved for gay couples and should be fully explored by any man or heterosexual couple wanting to unlock the full pleasure that a man's body is capable of.

Understanding Orgasms

We have discussed the female orgasm somewhat in this chapter so far, but in this section, we will look at it in a little more depth.

For a woman to reach orgasm, much of this is dependent on her mindset. She will need to feel comfortable being vulnerable in this space for her to reach her full arousal potential. She needs to reach this point in order for her to orgasm and in order for her to fully enjoy sex. For this reason, mindset and pleasure are very closely linked to a woman.

When the clitoris is rubbed in the right way, it will lead to orgasm, just like the penis of a man. Treating it like this can give both men and women insight into how it works and how to make the woman come. When stimulated physically with someone's fingers or a sex toy like a vibrator, this can lead to an orgasm for the woman. The clitoris is a structure that contains many nerve endings, which is what makes it so sensitive. When a woman is not aroused sexually, her clitoris is still there, but it will not be as enlarged as when she is horny.

A woman's vagina automatically swells when she is sexually aroused because of increased blood flow to her genitals, sort of like how your penis becomes erect when you get horny. What this means for you is that when your penis is inside of her, the walls of her vagina will tighten and swell as the blood flow increases, and you will feel this effect on your penis, resulting in added pleasure for you.

There are different types of multiple orgasms that a woman can achieve. Women are lucky in that they can have both back-to-back orgasms and blended orgasms. They are even able to have back-to-back blended orgasms in some cases! In this section, we will learn more about the different types of multiple orgasms.

We will now discuss blended orgasms. A blended orgasm is achieved when multiple different orgasms are achieved at the same time. This can be two different orgasms at the same time, or in some cases, even more than two! This type of orgasm leads to even more pleasure than a single orgasm and will lead the woman to feel more intense pleasure than ever before. During penetration, there is lots of opportunity for different types of female orgasms to occur. The two most common ways that a woman can reach orgasm are through her clitoris and through her G-spot. We will look at some ways that a woman can have both of these orgasms at the same time, as well as some other options for blended orgasms.

Any combination of these separate but simultaneous orgasms compounds to give the woman a mind-blowing, full-body, blended orgasm. This is especially so if the two locations of stimulation are a larger distance from each other- like the nipples and the clitoris for example. The best type of blended orgasm will vary from woman to woman, depending on her personal preferences and what her most sensitive erogenous zones are. Some of these zones include the clitoris, the anus, the G-Spot, and the nipples. Some women may have others as well, but this is largely dependent on the woman's body.

The first method is a clitoral orgasm during penetration. If the clitoris is stimulated while the man is penetrating the woman, she could have an orgasm through both her clitoris and her G-Spot at the same time. This type of multiple orgasms will make her feel pleasure like never before because these two places are extremely pleasurable even when achieved alone, so together it is a new level of orgasm! There are different ways that you can achieve this, but the most successful way is to penetrate her with your fingers while she rubs her clitoris at the same time. This way, you can feel your way around and stimulate her G-spot while she pleases herself. It may take some practice and will require a lot of communication, but eventually, you will both be able to time it so that she can have both of these orgasms at once. Another way that this can happen is while the man is thrusting his penis into her. While he is doing this, she can touch her clitoris using her fingers or a vibrator, or the man can stimulate her clitoris by using his fingers or a vibrator. Some specific positions will allow for the man's penis to reach the G-Spot when inside of her, and at the same time, the base of his penis or his pelvic region can rub her clitoris, causing both orgasms to happen at the same time. We will look at these specific positions later on in this book.

Another way that a woman can achieve a blended orgasm is through having both an anal and clitoral orgasm at the same time. This is similar to the blended orgasm in which the man is penetrating the woman with his penis while her clitoris is being stimulated, but in this case, it is done while you are having anal sex. The method will happen in a similar way to the vaginal penetration with clitoral stimulation, but the positions used will be slightly different as the positions used in this case would be ones that better allow for anal penetration while giving either the man or the woman free hands to stimulate the clitoris. Either the man or the woman can stimulate the woman's clitoris in a variety of anal sex positions using either their hands or a vibrating sex toy.

Another type of blended orgasm that is possible is a nipple orgasm and a clitoral orgasm. Not every woman is able to achieve a nipple orgasm, but if you are, then this could be a great option for a blended orgasm. If you are unsure whether you are able to reach orgasm through nipple stimulation alone, try this one in order to see if also your clitoris having stimulated leads to more sensitivity in your nipples as well.

One example of a position in which this type of blended orgasm can occur is the following. While you are sitting in a chair with your legs spread wide, your partner will get on his knees in front of you. He will then begin to give you oral sex on his knees. While licking and using his mouth to stimulate your clitoris, he will reach up to your breasts with his hands and massage your nipples with his fingers. Once he has done this for some time and began to please you, he will then switch and using his tongue. He will gently lick, suck and lick your nipples with his tongue, one at a time. While he does this, he will also move his hand down between your legs and stimulate your clitoris with his hand and fingers. Have him alternate back and forth using his mouth on your clitoris and then on your nipples. This will give you pleasure from both of these erogenous zones, and you will likely be able to experience a blended nipple and clitoral orgasm in this way, as long as he keeps stimulating both areas at the same time.

Not only can women have blended orgasms, but they can also have back-to-back orgasms. These orgasms occur one after the other and give the woman immense pleasure because she is able to keep coming again and again and again.

This type of repeated orgasm is only possible for women as the male body is unable to do this. This is because the male body has to wait for a refractory period after every orgasm. What this means is that there is an amount of time after an orgasm during which a man's body is unable to achieve an erection or have another orgasm. During this time, his body is recovering from the orgasm and needs this time to recuperate. The length of this period is different for every man, but it ranges between fifteen to thirty minutes in most males.

The great thing about the clitoris is that after orgasm, it may be very sensitive for a few minutes, but it maintains its "erection" and can be stimulated again a very short time after for a doubly pleasurable second orgasm. This can lead to a third and a fourth and beyond. This is why, as we discussed, it is beneficial to give a woman an orgasm during foreplay as it will increase her chances of orgasm during penetration because of how horny it will have made her. Sometimes, women's pleasure only builds after an initial orgasm instead of going back to zero before climbing again like a man's pleasure would have to. It is important for men to understand this difference because they can then take advantage of it and pleasure their woman to the fullest. While they await their refractory period, they can please their woman in a way that does not involve their penis, give her an orgasm, and then by the time this happens; he will be ready to get hard again and have a second round with her. All the while, she will become increasingly horny and pleased.

Another type of multiple orgasms that may be different from what you had in mind when hearing the words "multiple orgasms" is the simultaneous orgasm." This type of multiple orgasms is great for couples, especially long-term couples. This type of orgasm occurs when both the man and the woman are able to reach orgasm at the same time! The reason why this is great for long-term couples is that it takes practice and excellent communication during sex, but when mastered, it will unlock new levels of pleasure for both of you. When in a long-term relationship, one of the many positive things about having sex with each other is that you know just the right way to make each other orgasm. After having sex with each other so many times, you likely have this down to a science! This comes in handy here as you can use this knowledge to help you both orgasm at the same time.

Since you know how to get your partner to orgasm in mere minutes, you can touch each other exactly as you each like at the exact same time in order to reach orgasm simultaneously.

Now, this is a little more difficult than it sounds, but it is entirely possible. To do this, begin with the intention of orgasming together. Both of you will stimulate the other person's genitals in the best way you know, so you will have to figure out a position that allows for both of these ways at the same time. For example, if your partner can make you come very quickly by giving you oral sex while also massaging your testicles and you can make her come very quickly by playing with her clitoris just the right way, then you will have to find a position where you can do both of these at the same time. This position could be one where you are lying on your back on the bed, and she is straddling your chest, facing your feet. She will bend forward so that her mouth reaches your penis, and she will hold herself up with one of her arms on the bed. She can then use her other free hand to massage your testicles. You will then slide a hand between her legs and begin playing with her clitoris, and you can even use your other hand to slide your fingers into her vagina if she wishes.

When you begin, start out slow. This will require a lot of communication between the two of you. Begin pleasing each other and communicating your pleasure with moans or simple phrases like "that feels good" the entire time. When one of you gets close to reaching orgasm, tell the other person. If your partner tells you that they are close to coming, ease up on the pressure or the speed on her clitoris, for example, so that she does not come yet. When, and if you are also close to orgasm, let her know, and you can both continue to stimulate each other's genitals until you both orgasm together at the same time!

One of the benefits of this type of orgasm in a long-term relationship is that when you care about a person deeply, you find pleasure in seeing them pleased. When you please your partner to the point of orgasm, it usually will make you also feel pleasure. Because of this, as each of you comes closer to reaching orgasm, it will make the other person more aroused. For this reason, a long-term couple will be able to do this act of simultaneous orgasms with ease.

Understanding The Female Orgasm Potential
Female ejaculation is a well-disputed concept in modern discussions about sexuality. There is evidence though, that it is possible and actually quite common. While the term *female ejaculation* probably makes you think of something porn-related, it is something that can happen without theatrics and to a much lesser degree in your own sex life. Female ejaculation is often portrayed as a fountain of water spraying across the room; however, this is not the case in real life.

Female ejaculation does not have to occur, and, in many cases, it never does. It is sort of the icing on the cake or the cherry on top so to speak, but it is not necessary in order for the woman to be aroused or to achieve orgasm. Female ejaculation, commonly referred to as *squirting,* is different for every woman and does not have to involve a large amount of fluid like a male ejaculation. It also does not happen every time and does not only happen during orgasm. While it can happen at the time of orgasm, female ejaculation can also occur at any time during sex when the woman is extremely aroused. Thus, ejaculation can be a sign that the woman is feeling aroused regardless of whether she has reached orgasm yet or not. This is a good sign that indicates she is enjoying herself.

Ejaculation does not happen to every woman, but it can be something that can be practiced and learned if the woman would like to experience it. Some people become extremely turned on when they experience or witness female ejaculation, so if you or your partner feel that it would turn you both on, it is possible for the woman to begin trying to achieve this. For some people, it turns them on so much, even to the point of experiencing orgasm.

Female ejaculation has been linked to G-Spot stimulation, so the best way to achieve this is to have your partner stimulate your G-Spot with either his fingers, his penis, or a dildo.

What to Do First

The Kama Sutra text views sex as a spiritual act between two people that, with time, will increase a person's level of spirituality and sexual power. The book aims to help people to get in touch with their desires, which will aid them in reaching the full extent of their sexual power. It aims to liberate people in a sexual sense. These concepts were quite advanced for the time that the book was written, which is why this book is still so widely discussed to this day. Before you begin practicing the concepts of the Kama Sutra, it is important to understand this.

Lubrication

There are many different types of lubricants that you can use to make your sex glide easier and feel more pleasurable. The first type we will talk about is the synthetic lubricant. There are different types of these-water-based and silicone-based lubricants. The type of lubricant you choose will depend on what type of sex toy you are using and what your intended use is. I will go into more detail about the different types of lubrication below, but first, we will look at the benefits of using any lubrication during sex in general. Lubrication has been shown to have sex better in many ways, the first of which is that it makes all body parts glide better and slide easier, which means no painful dry skin on dry skin friction. Lubrication has also been shown to increase the intensity of both male and female orgasms. As I mentioned earlier, in order to have an orgasm vaginally for women or anally for either sex, constant rhythmic penetration is required. Lubrication makes this possible because of the ease of movement it allows for will help with maintaining a rhythm of penetration.

Lubrication can also be used for masturbation with sex toys or with hands and fingers alone for both men and women because it will make toys or fingers move and glide easier, which will lead to more pleasure. Lubrication will make both clitoral stimulation and penile stroking more pleasant because it will eliminate any skin on skin friction that would occur because of a lack of a condom or, in the case of male masturbation the lack of a female's natural vaginal lubrication to act as a lubricant on the penis.

Silicone-Based Lubricant

Silicone-based lube is the type of lube you would want to use if you want to have sex in the bathtub, shower, or any environment involving water since it won't rinse off when it becomes wet. If you are not using it to have sex in a wet environment, the other benefit about it is that it will usually only need to be applied once and will stay thick and doing its job for the duration of your session. This makes silicone-based lube a great choice for activities involving anal sex because it is thicker and longer-lasting than other forms of lubrication. When having anal sex of any sort, ample lubrication is required, and choosing the longer-lasting sort of lube will be best.

The drawback though, is that this type of lubrication is not very easy to clean. This is because it cannot be rinsed off by only using water. This variety of lubrication requires you to use soap and scrub it off of whatever you are cleaning it off of, like a penis or your vaginal area. Silicone-based lubricants aren't ideal on a silicone-based sex toy because it can cause the toy to break down more quickly over time than it normally would.

Water-Based Lubricant

Water-based lubricant is very easy to clean as it can be rinsed off of your body or your sex toys with water alone. The drawback though is that if you enjoy shower sex, bathtub sex, pool-sex, or any sex involving the water, it will wash away immediately and will not provide any lubrication as soon as it gets wet. This is also why this type of lubrication may need to be reapplied a few times in a session. If you do not have much shower or bathtub sex and you use silicone sex toys, then water-based lube would be good for you.

Oils

As an alternative, you can use oil as a lubricant. Oil is beneficial because it is so versatile in its uses. Oil can be used as a massage aid for some sensual foreplay massaging. It can be used without being washed off before oral sex because of its natural roots and its flavor that would not be terrible in your mouth. If you prefer something natural as a lubricant, then oil will likely be your choice. Many people will use coconut oil for this purpose. It can be used as an edible lubricant as it is often seen in cooking and smoothies. The one drawback to oil-based lubricants is that they can't be used with condoms because they will deteriorate the condom and cause it to break.

Gels

There are some gels that are made for sexual encounters that also can be used with versatility. There are some aloe vera scented gels that can be used both as a massage gel for foreplay and as lube for penetrative sex. If you live in a hot place or take this gel with you on vacation, it can also be an after-sun gel for burnt skin. This way, soothing your partner's sunburn could turn into quite the sensual and even sexual experience.

Kissing

There are 16 different kissing techniques outlined in the Kama Sutra. This means that you will never run out of new and interesting ways to show your partner love through kissing them.

- The Normal Kiss
- The Straight Kiss
- The Turned Kiss
- The Throbbing Kiss
- The Touching Kiss
- The Bent Kiss
- The Pressed Kiss
- The Gently Pressed Kiss
- Kiss of the Upper Lip
- A Clasping Kiss

- The Kiss that Kindles Love
- The Turning Away Kiss
- The Awakening Kiss
- Kiss of Showing Intention
- The Transferred Kiss
- The Demonstrative Kiss

Foreplay

Foreplay is generally treated as the time before penetrative sex, where there is some kissing, some touching, and some sensual whispers. What happens during foreplay? In the media, foreplay is often given a bad reputation, as it is portrayed as something that must be done for the woman's body to get ready for sex, or for the woman to feel comfortable enough to begin having sex. While some of this is true, sex is much more than the act of a penis in a vagina. Sex can last much longer than the time between when the man inserts his penis and when he reaches orgasm. The Kama Sutra recognizes that there should be much more importance placed on foreplay, which is why there are several sections of the text which talk about what you can do to share intimate moments with your partner before penetration.

Sex between couples is much more than what happens when the man is inside of the woman. Treating sex as much more than just a physical activity means that we must include all aspects of sex in our discussions about how to have a better sex life. This includes foreplay. That being said, if foreplay is considered part of sex, then the positions in which you engage in foreplay are sex positions.

In this section, we will look at foreplay as a special part of sex, and I will introduce some different techniques for foreplay that focus on your emotional connection and intimacy with your partner.

The Importance of Foreplay

Foreplay is important to ensure that you will be able to have comfortable sex. This is because the man will have to be erect enough, and the woman will have to be wet enough for sex to happen smoothly and without pain. This is the most practical reason that foreplay exists.

Further, foreplay gives you a chance to connect with your partner on an emotional level before you begin connecting physically in such a deep way. This time to connect with one another can make the difference between lovemaking and the physical act of sex. Connecting emotionally while connecting physically will lead to longer-lasting love and more passionate sex.

As we discussed above, foreplay is an important aspect of sex. This is especially true for women. This is because a woman needs to feel comfortable and relaxed to feel sexual pleasure. Foreplay serves to make a woman feel comfortable, letting her hair down, and being vulnerable. This is true whether she is in a long-term relationship or having a one-night stand.

The woman will need to feel comfortable being vulnerable in this space for her to reach her full arousal potential. Further, she needs to reach this point for her body to reach orgasm. Taking some time to set the mood before you have sex will go a long way in terms of a woman's ability to become and stay aroused. This will benefit both the man and the woman because the man will have more fun if the woman is comfortable. Setting the mood also shows the woman that you are concerned with her level of comfort in her surroundings and are invested in her pleasure. Her ability to have an orgasm will depend greatly on her level of ease.

Many times, foreplay involves some kind of stimulation of the genitals, whether it is by oral sex or using your hands. This gets you ready for sex, as your body will respond by becoming more and more aroused. Once in a full state of arousal, you can achieve successful penetration.

There are some benefits to using only your hands to please your partner. When using your hands, you can feel your way around their body. This will mean that you will know exactly what you are doing and where you are touching them at all times. You can control the pressure with which you hold or stroke the penis or rub the clitoris when you are using your hands. For the man, he can feel his way around inside of the woman so that he knows exactly where he is. This way, he can aim for a specific location such as her G-Spot or the deeper areas of her vagina. If he were using his penis, he would not have as much control or as much perception of where he was in relation to her G-Spot.

The other reason why foreplay is so important for the woman is that it is quite difficult for a woman's body to reach orgasm during penetrative sex. If the woman can orgasm during foreplay, she will enjoy penetrative sex much more!

Another reason that foreplay will allow a woman to get more enjoyment out of penetrative sex is the following; The time spent getting each other in the mood for sex will cause the woman's clitoris to become engorged. This is similar to a male erection. The benefit of this is that when you are having penetrative sex, and her clitoris is engorged, it will more easily make contact with the shaft of the man's penis or with some part of his body as he is thrusting into her. What this means is that it will be easier for her to get clitoral stimulation during penetrative sex is her clitoris becomes engorged during foreplay.

Kama Sutra Foreplay Techniques

The first technique we will look at is setting the mood. This may not seem of importance, but it is a very important part of pre-sex behavior that is often overlooked.

As a couple, it is more important to set the mood and environment for your sex than it would be if you were having casual sex or a one-night stand. In a relationship, you have moved past the casual awkwardness of those types of encounters and onto real lovemaking.

When setting the mood, our focus is on creating an environment free of distractions where you can both focus on each other without becoming side-tracked. Another focus is to create an environment that is relaxing and calm. This will allow you to get in touch with your sensations and your deeper feelings to embrace your pleasure and move in ways that feel good to you without your thoughts running too much and getting in the way of your body and its own needs. So, what do I do to set the mood and make the environment relaxing? Read on.

If you are having sex in your bedroom or your home, it is a space that is very familiar to both of you. This may mean that all of your regular distractions are present all over the place, including your phone, your computer, and your textbooks or your work maybe. You don't want these things staring at you from across the room, reminding you that you have to study all night or send a quick email after your orgasm is over, so try to keep the room as free of these things as possible. Maybe leave your phone and laptop in the kitchen or the office, and make sure you put it on silent!

Secondly, we want the environment to be relaxing. Get rid of the harsh lighting of your overhead bulbs and turn on a few lamps with a soft orange glow or light some candles. The candles may seem cheesy, but there is a reason that they became so closely associated with romance. You don't necessarily have to go so far as having rose petals and chocolates, but some candles will be a nice touch for any day of the week.

Setting the mood in this way will allow you both to breathe and focus on each other and yourselves. We all deserve to have some time with our partner and our bodies, where we enjoy the feeling of pleasure. Use this time with your partner as a way to de-stress and let yourself unwind. Have some fun. Now that the mood is set, the next stages of foreplay can begin.

When you begin foreplay, begin by feeling around between your partner's legs slowly. Pay attention to their face to see what areas are most sensitive and responsive to your touch. Remember, this could vary by the day, so what they liked yesterday may not be what they want today.

When you find the spot that is most responsive (or spots, plural), continue to stimulate it, gradually increasing your speed and pressure as they become more excited and hornier. Listen to their audible cues to tell you when you are hitting the right spot, the right speed, and the right pressure and continue with this in order to keep exciting them. They may reach orgasm, or this may lead to some other type of sex.

Being able to be sexually intelligent enough to know where to go, where to touch and how, and how to read the person and their cues takes time.

By stimulating a woman's clitoris, you can give her great pleasure if you know how to touch it the right way. During foreplay, try to give the woman an orgasm if possible. This will make her vagina extremely wet, which will lead to better penetrative sex.

How do you know when you have done enough foreplay? The answer to this is the woman's level of pleasure. It also depends on whether you are erect enough of course! If she has an orgasm during foreplay and you are both wanting to begin penetration, then that is an appropriate time to do so. If you want to extend foreplay even longer after she orgasms, by all means do so. If she does not orgasm during foreplay, you will know when you have spent enough time on this part of sex by how wet her vagina is and how ready she is to begin penetration. If she is getting very wet and is telling you she wants you to put your penis inside of her, it is safe to assume she is ready for you. If she is not too wet and she does not seem as passionate about the sex as she is when she is fully aroused, keep the foreplay going a little longer. You can use dirty talk to find out where she is at mentally as well. You can say something like, "do you want me to come into you?" "How wet are you?" or something of the sort. This will allow her to respond in a sexy way, telling you if she wants more in terms of foreplay, or if she is ready to take it to the next step.

Chapter 4: The Kama Sutra Massage Techniques

A great way to begin practicing Kama Sutra sex techniques is to start with a massage. Every couple can have a quick session of sexual intercourse, but this will not provide you with all of the potential benefits that the Kama Sutra contains. By starting with a sensual massage, you and your partner will share intimate moments together, which will have sex that much better once you get to that stage in this book.

The Kama Sutra Classic Massage Technique

The Kama Sutra talks about massages, including the best places to give massages and some techniques for doing so.

Sometimes, giving your partner a massage will lead to penetrative sex, and sometimes it will not. Aside from being part of foreplay, a massage can also be a relaxing gesture of love. Giving your partner a massage at the end of the day is a great way to get intimate with each other.

If you have massage oil, that is a great addition to any massage, but if not, you can use coconut oil. If you don't have either of those, you can use something like lotion to lubricate your hands and avoid skin to skin friction. Warm your hands before you start massaging them so that it feels nice and doesn't send a chill down their spine when you first make contact.

You can let your partner choose what type of massage they'd like- foot, head, back, shoulder, etc. Instruct them to lie in a comfortable position for their massage. Once you have lubricated your hands, put your hands on them lightly. Then you can begin to massage them gently.

The touch of a massage from a lover gives a person a sense of being cared for. It is a great way to deepen your bond. A massage is a great way to show your partner that you care about making them feel good.

After you have massaged their upper body or their feet, begin kissing their body where you just massaged it and then progress to kissing them on the lips. Let this encounter naturally progress, and let your bodies guide you. You can gradually move into touching each other in new areas, and maybe you will even begin touching each other's genitals, though that leads us to the next section of this chapter.

Eventually, all of this massaging could lead to sex, but it doesn't have to. We will discuss this in more detail below.

The Kama Sutra Erotic Massage Versus the Kama Sutra Classic Massage

Above, we saw an example of a classic Kama Sutra massage. This massage technique does not involve sex or massaging of the genitals. This style of massage involves the person's entire body or any specific location that they would like you to focus on. This kind of massage can be done anywhere and does not necessarily require either of you to remove your clothes.

Beginning with a relaxing massage such as the classic massage will help you and your partner to get into a relaxed and connected state of mind. Once you have finished with the classic massage, you may feel the urge to touch your partner and massage them in other places. This brings us to the erotic massage.

An erotic massage is a massage that involves the touching and massaging of a person's genitals. This leads to pleasurable sensations, but not necessarily to orgasm. An erotic massage can lead to orgasm, though that is not the sole intention.

Erotic massages can be given to both men and women, and they will lead to pleasure and relaxation. You can find a sample technique for a female and a male erotic massage outlined below.

The Benefits of Both

In this section, we are going to look at some of the many benefits that massages can provide you with.

- Relaxing

A massage, regardless of which type, is a relaxing way to unwind with your partner.

- Pleasurable

Massages are pleasurable, whether they are massages of the body or erotic massages. They bring a sense of pleasure in the form of human touch.

- Can be Done Man to Woman or Woman to Man

Massages are able to be done by anyone, to anyone. This makes them a great option for any kind of couple or relationship.

- Can be Done Anytime, Anyplace

Since you don't necessarily have to be naked, a massage can be done anytime, anywhere. This makes it a great option for any couple.

The Female Erotic Massage

This type of massage is an erotic massage, which is called the *yoni massage*. A yoni massage involves the woman's entire vaginal area, which is called the *vulva*. The vulva is a broad term for the vaginal area, which includes the clitoris, the large and small labia, the vagina, and the general areas around them. This area is full of nerve endings, so a woman can feel great pleasure from a massage in this location.

A Yoni Massage is done to open up the woman to her sexuality, her pleasure, and her sexual desires. As a partner, you can perform this type of massage for your female partner to unlock her hidden sexual energy and help her to get in touch with it. For this reason, this massage is a great addition to foreplay, though it can also be done independently of sex.

This massage can be done in a variety of ways, such as in a bathtub, in a jacuzzi, in bed or on the floor. The most important factor here is that the woman is feeling comfortable and relaxed, and the environment will play a big role in this.

To help the woman relax before her massage, begin by setting the ambiance. Ensure that you remove distractions so that she can focus on her pleasure.

You can prepare your hands in the same way that you lubricated and warmed your hands for the classic massage, but be sure that you are using lubricant for this type of massage.

Begin by having the woman breathe deeply and focus on her body. Let her know that she can begin getting in touch with any sensations she is having.

Begin by slowly and gently massaging around her entire vulva and her clitoral area. The key to this type of massage is to move very slowly and with intention. Begin to massage her clitoris slowly and do so without the intention of making her come. You are instead trying to give her subtle pleasure. Massage around her entire vulva slowly, including her labia. Do this for a few minutes, being sure to focus on the entire area and not just her clitoris.

When ready, and using lube, slide one finger into her vagina. Begin to gently massage the inside of her vagina.

By lifting your fingers towards the front of her body, you will find the location of her G-spot.

Encourage her to express herself vocally and to release any sounds she naturally makes as a result of this massage. Move your fingers in a circular motion slowly and with your other hand, massage her pelvic area, her vulva, and clitoris. Doing this serves to connect the inner with the outer.

Continue to massage her in this way and let the experience unfold with no end goal in mind. Let her know that if her body reaches orgasm, she should not fight it. If she doesn't reach orgasm, she can simply enjoy the pleasure that the massage is providing her with. As discussed earlier, this massage is intended to reconnect a woman with her pleasure and allow her to focus on herself and her body, so an orgasm is not necessary.

After this massage, she will feel more in touch with her body. If penetrative sex ensues, both of you will feel increased levels of pleasure, and your orgasms will be more intense because of how engorged and activated her vagina and clitoris will be after having been massaged.

The Male Erotic Massage

There are several different options for providing your male partner with an erotic massage. Firstly, you can massage their testicles. This is less likely to lead to orgasm than a penis massage, so it can be a great way to get a man relaxed and in the mood.
Another form of erotic massage for men, which is discussed in the Kama Sutra, is the penis massage. This type of massage can be tricky, as it could lead to orgasm quite quickly. The effectiveness of this massage will depend on the man's ability to last as his penis is being massaged.

The third variety of massage is the prostate massage. Since this type of massage requires the man's partner to insert a finger into his anus, some couples may be less comfortable with this type of erotic massage. If you do wish to try this kind of massage, it can be very pleasing for the man. The *prostate* is a small gland located inside a man's body between the base of his penis and his anus. It is accessed through the anus. This type of massage is similar to anal sex, but it is not the same, as the goals are different, and so is the technique. Keep in mind that this type of massage will require you to use lots of lube for maximum comfortability. Once your fingers are well-lubricated, you can slide a finger or two inside of the man's anus very slowly. As we discussed previously, you will have to go slow so as not to shock the anus into closing tightly. You will need to work your way in gradually. Once in, you will be able to find the prostate by feeling around on the upper (front) wall of the rectum for a small lump that is rough in texture a few inches deep. Once you have found it, you can begin to gently massage it. You can move your fingers in circles and apply light pressure to it. This massage has the potential to feel quite pleasurable for the man. Communicate while the massage is occurring in order to give him the most pleasure possible.

You can perform this type of massage in a number of different positions. The man could be lying down while you straddle his legs, he could be on his hands and knees while you sit or kneel behind him, he could lie across your lap while you sit on a bed, or you could do any position that is comfortable for you.

This massage does not need to lead to orgasm; at least that is not the goal. If it happens, that is fine; however, the aim of this massage is just to provide a relaxing and pleasurable experience for him.

That is the extent to which we will discuss the prostate massage, and we will now focus on the testicle massage. This type of massage is the most common and the most successful for relaxation and pleasure.

You can perform the testicle massage in several different positions. The man could be lying down on the bed, he could be reclining in a chair, be in a sitting position, or you any other position that is comfortable for him. This massage does not need to lead to orgasm- that is not the goal. If it happens, that is fine; however, the aim of this massage is simply to provide a relaxing and pleasurable experience for the man.

Remember from our discussion of the classic massage, if you have massage oil, that is preferable for this type of massage, but if not, you can use coconut oil. If you don't have either of those, you can use a sexual lubricant to lubricate your hands and avoid skin to skin friction. This is especially important when massaging the testicles. Before you touch him, warm your hands by rubbing them together. This will ensure that it feels nice and that it doesn't shock his testicles if you touch them with cold hands.

Begin by cupping your warm hand around his testicles. Gently move your hand in a circular motion. Be sure not to squeeze them too tightly, especially as you are beginning. Allow the testicles to warm up and relax. Massage them in a circular motion and apply gentle pressure to them. You can incorporate your second hand to provide him with extra sensation.

If he can handle it, you can gently touch his penis as you massage his testicles. If he becomes too erect and is about to reach orgasm, focus solely on the testicles. Massage the area around his testicles, including his inner thighs and his lower butt.

Let this massage flow and see where it takes you. Encourage him not to hold back and to let out any sounds that may find themselves escaping his mouth. Try to help him last as long as he can as you massage him.

After completing this massage, you may find that he is extremely horny, and this may lead to sex. If so, there is no problem with that. Enjoy yourselves and the increased pleasure that will come after such a sensual experience together.

Chapter 5: Kama Sutra Sex Positions

Today in pop culture, the Kamasutra's 64 sex positions are often discussed, making it seem like this book is a secret guide to penetrative sex. By this point in the book, you know that this is untrue. In this chapter, we are going to begin looking at some of the sex positions contained within the Kama Sutra to give you an idea of what exactly this book says about sex.

You may have actually performed one or two of these Kama Sutra sex positions without even knowing that they came from this ancient book. In this chapter, we are going to begin our discussion of the Kama Sutra sex positions by looking at the easiest and simplest sex positions that it contains. In the chapters that follow, we are going to look at Kama Sutra positions for intimacy, as well as some of the more advanced sex positions.

Many people wish to try these sex positions for themselves, and they have become quite popular in the mainstream media today. Many variations can be found, which have come as a result of tweaking the original positions of the Kama Sutra. People always push the envelope when it comes to sexual intercourse and physical pleasure, and many novel sex positions have come about as a result. Maybe you will recognize one or two of these!

Easy Kama Sutra Sex Positions

We are going to begin by looking at some of the easier Kama Sutra sex positions. These positions can be done by any couple, regardless of your strength or flexibility.

The Reverse Cowgirl

This position is quite a classic position, though it is one of the positions included in the book of Kama Sutra. This position is great for the female orgasm, as it allows the woman to take control since she is on top.

To get into this position, the man will lie down on his back on the bed. The woman will straddle him, but instead of facing his head, she will face his lower body, as depicted above. From here, the woman can lift her body up and down, using her legs at the speed and depth that feels best. She can also thrust at the angle that she enjoys the most, and she can feel the pleasure build as she moves her body. The man can sit back and relax, as the woman rides him sensually.

Below, you can see another variation of the Reverse Cowgirl Position, in which the woman opens up her body to allow for clitoral stimulation at the same time as penetration. In this variation, the woman will lie back so that she is lying on top of the man, facing away from him- his penis still inside of her. She can plant one of her hands back onto the bed to help hold herself up, while the other hand stimulates her clitoris. She can also use a vibrator on her clitoris in this position.

The Congress of a Dog

This position is called *The Congress of a Dog*. This is a position in which the man and woman are intended to emulate two animals having sex. In this case, they are intended to act as a male dog mating with a female dog. This is similar to the position above, but in this case, this position can be likened to the modern *Doggy Style* position.

This position is a favorite among men and women alike. Both women and men can get intense pleasure from this position because the angles at which their genitals come together creates harmonic pleasure for both parties.

To get into position, the woman gets on her hands and knees on the bed (or couch or floor, this position works anywhere really), and the man kneels behind her. He takes his erect penis and enters her vagina. He starts by slowly sliding it in and gradually begins getting faster and deeper. He does this by thrusting his hips and can control the pace in this way. He grabs onto her hips for a stronger thrust and pulls her body towards his to get himself deeper into her with each thrust. In this position, he has a view of her entire backside and can see it shake and bounce with each movement, making him hornier and hornier. He can talk dirty to her and grab her butt cheeks from here.

Doggy style is a position that women can get a lot of pleasure from. It is no surprise it is most often the favorite position, especially among young people, of both genders. Because of the curve of the man's erect penis and the angle at which it enters into the woman's vagina, her G-spot will likely be stimulated with each thrust. This G-spot stimulation means that it will be very likely that she will reach an orgasm from penetration. G spot stimulation can make a woman feel such intense full-body pleasure for quite a long time before she actually reaches an orgasm. Hitting her G-spot will continue to feel amazing for both the woman and man until finally, one or both of them cannot wait any longer, and ultimate pleasure is reached.

The Supported Congress

This position is a variety of the standing position, but it can be done with more ease than some of the other standing varieties.

To get into this position, the man stands in front of a wall with the woman standing in front of him, facing him. The woman lifts one knee and wraps her leg around one of the man's legs. The man can then slide his penis into her vagina; her leg raised to allow for deeper penetration and easier access. In standing positions, it may be more difficult to get the penetration right away, but with some maneuvering and adjustments because of height differences, you will eventually get into a comfortable rhythm.

This position is a midway point to another Kamasutra position called The Suspended Congress, where the woman has both legs up, and the man is holding them both under her knees and thrusting into her while holding her weight up. This position is quite difficult for the man, but if achieved, it can lead to very deep penetration. The Supported Congress is a great place to start if you want to eventually try it with both legs up, as it is quite similar.

The Mare's Position

This Kama Sutra position is more of a sexual technique than a sex position itself. This sexual technique has the potential to change your sex life forever!

In this position, the man sits with his legs stretched out in front of him and his arms back, supporting his weight on the bed. The woman straddles him, facing away from him and lowers herself down onto his erect penis. Once inside of her, the woman uses her vaginal muscles to apply and release pressure on the man's penis, almost as if she is milking it. This makes for very pleasurable sensations on both the man's penis and the woman's vagina. This creates more stimulation on the man's penis, and also stronger sensations for the woman's vagina. This also strengthens her vaginal muscles, which in time will lead to stronger and more pleasurable orgasms for the woman!

Afternoon Delight

Afternoon Delight is a nice position to try on a quiet Sunday after a long work week when you are both feeling tired and want a bit of lazy sex. You can start this position off with some lazy hand and finger play and then progress it to penetration in the same position if you are already cuddling and don't want to move around too much. This position is optimal for stoners and sleepyheads.

The man lies down on his side, his erect penis poking out in front of him. The woman lies on her back at a 90-degree angle to the man's body, halfway down near his genitals. She then bends her knees, lifts her legs, and drapes them over the man's side, sliding her vagina towards him, so it is close to his penis. He can move forward to meet her and slide his penis in her vagina. The woman can lie back and relax while the man thrusts his hips. This position can be done while you watch a tv show, while you are reading or while you are both half-asleep and want a little bit of Afternoon Delight. If this inspires you to try something more involved once you get into the mood, you can easily transition to Missionary or Doggy Style from here.

The Lap Position

This next position is another that is best for male pleasure and the male orgasm. This position requires strength on the part of the man and the woman and is quite an athletic position, but this is why it is called an advanced sex position. Be careful when trying this one.

To get into position, the man will sit upright in a comfortable chair or on the edge of a bed with his feet planted on the floor. The woman will climb onto his lap and wrap her legs around behind the man or stick them straight out past him. Then, the man can insert his penis into the woman's vagina. From here, the woman will lean back until she is lying straight back, and her body is flat. While she does this, the man will have to hold onto her at her hips or her lower back, depending on your height variations. The man in this position will perform a combination of thrusting his hips into the woman from a seated position and pulling her onto his penis repeatedly. A high amount of upper body strength is required on the part of the man in this position. Place some pillows on the floor underneath the woman when trying this position, just in case. The woman can hold onto the man's arms for support as well here.

This position is great for the male's pleasure because it allows him to control the speed and depth of thrusting.

The Ascending Position

This position allows the woman to take full control of both her body and the man's penis and is good for women who have some trouble reaching orgasm in other sexual positions. The man takes a passive role in this position, with the woman's weight on top of him, which can be a huge turn-on. He can lie back and watch her take control and enjoy the pleasure he is getting from his penis inside of her and from watching the woman gyrate and find pleasure on top of him.

The man lies down on his back on the bed; he can prop up his head on a pillow if he wants a better view of the woman. She sits cross-legged on top of his genital area, her legs crossed over his waistline. She holds onto his penis and puts it into her vagina. She can wait to do this after oral or after giving him a handjob first, or she can get right to the penetration, depending on if they have already done foreplay prior to this. Once he is inside of her, she can lean back and rest her hands on his legs for support if needed. From here, she grinds her hips and can control her hip angles and control the speed of thrusting. In this leaned back position, her clitoris is perfectly accessible to be stimulated with her own hand. The man will be too far to do this for her as he is lying down, and her legs are holding his body down. The restriction of his movement by his naked woman will be sure to make the man so horny and frustrated that his penis will be rock hard. She can change the angle of her hips to reach G-spot stimulation by the man's penis. She may even be able to reach both clitoral and G-spot orgasms at the same time from this position.

The Cross Position

This position is similar to another position of the Kama Sutra, the Half-Pressed Position. If you like this one, you are sure to like the Half-Pressed Position too.

The woman lies on her back with one leg extended straight into the air. The man kneels in front of her, straddling her leg that is extended on the bed and holds onto her other leg, which is in the air. He can then move his body forward between her two legs until he is close enough to insert his penis into her vagina. He can hold her legs spread with his body, straddling one of them and placing the other one on his shoulder. By doing this, his hands will be free so that he can play with her clitoris, massage her breasts, rubbing his hands up and down her body or whatever they please. They can talk dirty to each other while looking at each other in the eyes and tell each other what they want to be done to them or what feels good.

Chapter 6: The Kama Sutra and Intimacy

For a book written so long ago, it is still quite relevant in terms of its discussions on ways to achieve intimacy and how to treat your partner well in the bedroom. In this chapter, we are going to talk about the best Kama Sutra sex positions for intimacy and what the Kama Sutra can teach you about improving the level of intimacy in your relationship or marriage.

What Is Intimacy?

Intimacy is very important between two people when part of a couple, especially in the bedroom. Intimacy is what brings you close and keeps you close. For this reason, we are going to address intimacy in this chapter before moving onto the rest of the concepts related to sex, sex positions, and techniques for you and your partner. Firstly, we will look at what intimacy means and the different types of intimacy that exist.

There are different types of intimacy, and here I will outline them for you before digging deeper into the intimacy that exists between couples. Intimacy, in a general sense, is defined as mutual openness and vulnerability between two people. There are different ways in which you can give and receive openness and vulnerability in a relationship. Intimacy does not have to include a sexual relationship (though it can); therefore, it is not only reserved for romantic relationships. Intimacy can also be present in other types of close relationships like friendships or family relationships. Below, I will outline the different forms of intimacy.

- Emotional Intimacy

Emotional intimacy is the ability to express oneself maturely and openly, leading to a deep emotional connection between people. Saying things like "I love you" or "you are very important to me" are examples of this. It is also the ability to respond maturely and openly when someone expresses themselves to you by saying things like "I'm sorry" or "I love you too." This type of open and vulnerable dialogue leads to an emotional connection. For a deep emotional connection to form, there must be a mutual willingness to be vulnerable and open with one's deeper thoughts and feelings. This is where this type of emotional intimacy comes from.

- Physical Intimacy

Physical intimacy is the type that most people think of when they hear the term "intimacy," and it is the kind that we will be most concerned with in this book, as it is the type of intimacy that includes sex and all activities related to sex. It also involves other non-sexual types of physical contact, such as hugging and kissing. Physical intimacy can be found in close friendships or familial relationships where hugging and kisses on the cheek are common, but it is most often found in romantic relationships.

Physical intimacy is the type of intimacy involved when people are trying to make each other orgasm. Physical intimacy is almost always required for orgasm. Physical intimacy doesn't necessarily mean that you are in love with the person you are having sex with; it just means that you are doing something intimate with another person in a physical way.

It is also possible to be intimate with yourself, and while this begins with the emotional intimacy of self-awareness, it also involves the physical intimacy of masturbation and physical self-exploration. I define sexual, physical intimacy of the self as being in touch with the parts of yourself physically that you would not normally be in touch with. If you are a woman, your breasts, your clitoris, your vagina, and your anus. If you are a man, your testicles, your penis, your anus. Being able to be physically intimate with yourself allows you to have more fulfilling sex, more fulfilling orgasms, and a more fulfilling overall relationship with your body. We will discuss this in more detail later on in this book. Allowing someone to be physically intimate with you in a sexual way is also an emotionally intimate experience, regardless of your relationship with the person. Being in charge of your own body while it is in the hands of another person is very important, and this is why masturbation is such a key element to physical intimacy.

You can think of physical intimacy as something that breaks the barrier of personal space. By this definition, this includes touching of any sort, but especially sexual intercourse, kissing touching, and anything else of a sexual nature. When you are having sex with anyone, regardless of whether you have romantic feelings for them or not, you are having a physically intimate relationship with them. The difference between a relationship that involves physical intimacy alone and no other forms of intimacy and a romantic relationship is that a romantic relationship will also involve emotional intimacy, shared activities and intellectual intimacy is that a deep and lasting romantic relationship will need to include all of these forms of intimacy at once. In this book, we are going to focus on how all of these types of intimacy come together to create a successful and deep romantic relationship between two people in love. We are going to begin by taking the next section to discuss how to maintain and increase the levels of intimacy in your relationship.

The Importance of Intimacy

Feeling awkward when it comes to talking about intimacy is one of the most human experiences a person can have. Sometimes, we fall into a sexual rut with someone, and then we realize that the fiery passion that used to burn at the base of your tummy has dimmed. The way to remedy this is to work on your intimacy.

When it comes to a long-term relationship, you likely have reached a high level of intimacy, and this is often what makes your sex life so rewarding. While you can achieve physical pleasure from having sex with anyone, or from masturbating alone, the connection that you feel when having sex with someone whom you are emotionally intimate with will lead your physical body to be in harmony with your emotions and this leads to great levels of both physical and emotional pleasure, which is exactly where the term "making love" comes from.

When you care about another person deeply, you care about bringing them pleasure in a variety of forms; sexual pleasure is one of them. When you bring two people together who are genuinely invested in the pleasure of each other, this forms a beautiful sexual bond full of pleasure in every sense. This is why intimacy is important in sex and why sex with intimacy is not only a physical act but also an emotional experience.

The Kama Sutra and Intimacy

The Kama Sutra has quite a few things to say about intimacy and how to maintain and restore it. As I mentioned, the Kama Sutra is a guide to love and to enjoy a pleasurable life with your partner. The Kama Sutra can serve as a guide for a long-term relationship or a marriage to keep sex interesting and to try new forms of intimacy. By keeping your relationship new and different, it will keep you both interested in what is to come, which will keep you both engaged in your relationship with one another.

The Kama Sutra text views sex as a spiritual act between two people that, with time, will increase a person's level of spirituality and sexual power. The book aims to help people to get in touch with their desires, which will aid them in reaching the full extent of their sexual power. It aims to liberate people in a sexual sense. These concepts were quite advanced for the time that the book was written, which is why this book is still so widely discussed to this day. Even though it was written so long ago, this book is still quite relevant for couples who wish to improve their relationship or their level of intimacy.

Sex is one part of a romantic relationship, but there are so many other aspects to achieving deep emotional closeness with another person, which can be learned through reading the Kama Sutra. The rest of this book will focus on discussing many of the benefits of the Kama Sutra and the ways that it can help you increase your level of intimacy with your partner.

For example, the Kama Sutra states that taking a bath together is a great way to build intimacy in a relationship.

Taking a bath together is a nice way to unwind after a long day and spend some time together on self-care. Doing self-care together is actually quite intimate, as this is something usually reserved for our time alone.

Relaxing in a warm bath, either with bubbles or without, is a good way to set a mood. Sitting together in the closeness of a bathtub with the steam and the cleanliness will get you both in touch with your own bodies, but also in touch with their body. While this doesn't have to lead to sex, it can be a type of foreplay whether you intend for it to be or not. You may get in the bath together to spend some time to relax and share a few kisses. This may turn to making out and progress to much more. You may also get into the bath together to get yourselves in the mood for love and get naked while slowly easing into the sex. In Kamasutra, it is said that washing someone else's hair is a very intimate act. This may not be something that you have thought of before, or may not be something you are interested in. I assure you; it will lead to a greater level of intimacy with your partner if you give it a chance. When these acts of self-care that are usually done in private are shared with our partner, it can create magical moments of connection.

When you get into the bath, you can give each other head massages, back massages, or soap each other up. Begin kissing and making out and gliding your hands over your partner's wet body. Start with their back and arms and face. Let your desires take over both of you. As mentioned above, setting the mood like this will have you both focused on pleasure and touch and forgetting about all of your responsibilities and stressors in no time. This is good! We want to be focused when we have sex as a couple. Begin with one of you lathering the other with soap and shampoo in a slow and caring fashion. Rinse them off in the same way, taking care of their special needs and routines. Then, do the same the other way around. Take your time with this and enjoy the moment. You can do this as an act leading up to making love, or simply as a caring gesture for each other before bed.

It won't necessarily lead here, but a positive aspect of bathing together is that you will both be naked already for wherever you decide to take your sex from here. You will also both be clean, so any type of oral sex can be done without wondering when your partner last showered. As we all know, when we get comfortable with someone, we tend to put less into our image as we don't feel the need to impress them anymore!

How to Increase and Maintain Intimacy

Shared interests and activities are one of the forms of intimacy. This form of intimacy is less well-known, but it is also considered a form of intimacy. When you share activities with another person that you both enjoy and are passionate about, this creates a sense of connection. For example, when you cook together or travel together. These shared experiences give you memories to share, and this leads to bonding and intimacy (openness and vulnerability).

Being able to be vulnerable and open with your emotions is a requirement for intimacy. It is necessary to share oneself with the other person in a relationship. This mutual sharing of yourselves is what will lead to intimacy in the first place or an increase in intimacy.

Sometimes in a long-term relationship, you become so comfortable with each other that you don't have to communicate as much as you used to since you know each other so well. The key here is to continue communicating, even if you think the other person knows what you are thinking or feeling without you having to say it. By doing this, you keep the lines of communication open in your relationship. This avoids any chance of miscommunication or misunderstanding that would be perpetuated by a lack of communication. By having misunderstandings go unresolved, this could lead to resentment and an overall breakdown in communication, which can reduce levels of intimacy in the relationship.

This intimacy and vulnerability include being able to communicate about your desires- be they sexual desires or any other sort of desires. By sharing these with your partner, you will be able to ensure that they know how to please you in every sense of the word. This also leads to boundaries being set and upheld, since your desires include things you are comfortable and okay with, and this conversation will often lead to things which you are not okay with.

By learning these things about your partner, you can begin to work together to ensure each person's intimacy needs are met. For example, if your number one intimacy preference is for emotional intimacy and your partner likes to show their love in physical ways, you can discuss how they can begin to be more vocal about their love for you, and you can be more receptive to their physical displays of affection.

Putting these things out on the table for discussion is the best way to learn about each other. You can never stop learning about your partner, and this will only strengthen your relationship.

It is important to communicate about your needs for intimacy regularly since people will grow and change over the course of a relationship. Especially in a long-term relationship, being aware of when a person's intimacy needs change is important to maintaining a good level of intimacy.

Another way that romance is shown and received is through gestures and gifts. This is probably the first thing you think of when you hear the term "romance" for example, bringing your partner flowers after they have a long day, or drawing them a bath when you know they are feeling stressed out. These gifts and gestures are ways of communicating that don't involve words. When you are in a long-term relationship, it is important to be able to show your love and adoration in ways other than saying "I love you," and gestures are a great way to do this. If you and your partner have gotten into a routine way of living with each other, try to spice things up by offering to cook them dinner or by changing something up in order to show them your feelings and bring about some extra romance. This will help you to feel connected in new ways and will keep your spark alive, even if you are extremely comfortable with one another.

Kama Sutra Sex Positions for Intimacy

The Lotus

Arguably the most intimate position of them all is The Lotus. The Lotus position is most intimate because of the closeness of your entire bodies, infinitely pressed against each other at all points from head to toe, while being face to face.

The man sits on the bed cross-legged, his torso upright. His penis is erect and ready to get it on. The woman climbs on top of him and sits in his lap, wrapping her arms and legs around him. He holds her by wrapping his arms around her as well. With some shifting, they slide his penis inside of her. In this position, both people will be grinding more than they will be thrusting or humping. This is also what makes it so intimate. Grinding face to face while she is sitting on his lap with him inside of her, that is about as intimate as it gets.

In this position, you will not be doing any crazy thrusting, so it is ideal for a steamy make-out session, as your mouths will be so close that you can feel each other's breath the entire time. You can look into each other's eyes and whisper sweet nothings to them as you share this intimate experience.

The Position of Indra's Wife

To get into this position, the woman will lie down on her back, and she will bring her thighs to her sides.

She will bend her knees so that her legs are bent at her sides. This opens up her entire vaginal area for intercourse. The man will lie on top of her and enter her from the front.

This position may take practice due to the flexibility is requires from the woman, but if she can accomplish this, it will be greatly pleasurable for her. This position opens up the woman to receive the man, which will result in deeper penetration, and thus, greater pleasure for both of them.

Half-Pressed Position

This position is another midpoint to a more difficult Kamasutra position requiring a lot of flexibility, but this one is quite good even at this midway point! The woman's legs are spread wide, and so it is very pleasurable for both of them.

The woman lies down on her back with her man kneeling in front of her. She stretches one leg straight out past him, besides his body and with the other leg, she bends her knee and places her foot on his chest. From here, he enters her vagina. The woman can move her hips up or down to give varying amounts of pressure to the man's penis for added pleasure for him. The stretching of her leg opens her clitoris up to potentially be stimulated by the base of his penis when he thrusts his hips and penetrates deeply into her. Having one foot planted on his chest keeps her legs open wide with every one of his thrusts in order to allow for deep penetration and clitoral stimulation.

The Hinge Position

You may have tried this position before, but may not have known that it was a Kamasutra position. This position is a spin on doggy style, so if you are a big fan of the classic Doggy Style position, give this one a try next time you want to experiment with something new!

The man kneels on the bed with one knee down as usual, and the other leg propped up at a 90-degree angle. The woman is on all fours in front of the man, supporting her weight on her forearms. The man slides his penis into the woman's vagina from behind. Both the woman and the man are able to control the depth and speed from this position as the woman can thrust herself back onto his penis, and the man can thrust his hips forward. With one knee bent, the man has more control over his thrusts and can hold onto his woman's hips for a quicker speed if they want a deeper thrust and a faster and more rough sex session. This is one of those positions where it makes a quick thrusting speed easy because his knee is propped up.

The Closed Door

This position is similar to the missionary position in that both people are lying down face-to-face, and the man is on top. The difference, however, and what makes this an advanced position is that the woman will keep her legs shut tightly the entire time. The man's penis can be inserted while her legs are open, and then once it is in, she will close her legs. What this does is constrict her vagina and make the canal tighter for the man's penis. In addition to this, if she is aroused, her vagina will be engorged, and the canal will be tighter already. Because of this, the man's penis will be hugged closely as it slides in and out of her, and this will make for extra pleasure for him.

The Lock

To get into this position, the woman will lean back and relax on the bed, getting ready to receive her partner. Her partner will then approach her from the front, placing her legs on his shoulders and lifting her buttocks onto his thighs, as he will be sitting on his legs, which are bent behind him. The woman will lift her upper body slightly so that she can wrap her arms around her partner's shoulders or his neck. The man will support the woman's lower back, and then he can thrust into her from his sitting position, and he can use his arms to lift and lower her body onto his penis.

Variation of the Yawning Position

Have you ever heard of the term 'balls deep'? Have you ever wanted to try it?

The Yawning Position creates the deepest possible penetration of any sexual position. In the classic yawning position, the woman puts her legs in the air and spreads her legs with her knees straight, forming a 'V' shape. The man kneels in front of her and puts his penis inside her from the front. This creates an intense sensation for both partners.

The variation of The Yawning Position that we are going to look at can begin when the woman is fully aroused and wet. The woman lies on her back and lifts her legs into the air with her knees straight. The man lies on top of her in a missionary-like position. She places her straight legs on the man's shoulders. He can then enter her vagina with his erect penis and thrust his hips forward for the deepest penetration. As I said, this position makes for the deepest possible vaginal penetration of any sexual position, and if the woman can manage it, she can slide her legs to the outer edges of the man's shoulders which will make for maximum depth of penetration as her legs will be as far spread as possible.

The Standing Behind Position

In this position, the woman will stand facing a wall and will plant her hands on the wall in front of her. She will then bend her knees so that she can spread her legs. The man will come up behind and below her and come into her from behind. He can grab onto her hips or her shoulders so that he has something to hold onto, and he can use this to thrust deeper into her. This position is good in the shower or in any room of the house as having the woman planting her hands on the wall is both hot and safe when it comes to shower sex. This would be especially useful in the tight space of a stand-up shower. Just be sure to use lots of lubrication!

The Crab Position

In this position, the woman will lie on her back, and she will cross her legs. Then, she will hold her legs to her stomach. The man can assist by holding her legs there while he lies on top of her and enters her from the front. This position is quite intimate as it requires the man and woman to work together to hold her body in this posture. They are face to face while doing so, which makes it quite an intimate experience.

The Raised Feet Position

This position needs a little bit of flexibility, but it is also a sort of a stretch, so if you ease into it you should be able to reach it in a few minutes after your body is warmed up.

The woman lies on her back and brings her knees to her chest, wrapping her arms around them, her body forming a small ball shape. The man kneels near her buttocks and enters her vagina from a kneeling position in front of her. Her vagina will be quite easily accessible because her legs are lifted at her chest. If the flexibility is there, the man can now lean forward with his upper body, and with his own chest, he can hold her legs to her chest for her so that her hands are free. With her free hands, she can hold the back of his neck, pull his hair, or caress his face, depending on what direction you want to go with this sexual encounter. From here, the man's penis can very easily meet the woman's G-spot because of its curve, and this will make for an intense orgasm for both parties. The restriction of movement paired with the extreme closeness of their bodies is sure to make for some pent-up arousal that has no other way to be released than through a full-body orgasm.

The Waterfall

This position requires lots of trust between the woman and the man. The waterfall is a position in which the man has complete control. The man will begin by sitting in a chair with his feet on the floor. The woman will climb onto his lap and insert his penis into her. She can wrap her legs around his waist. Then, slowly she will lean all the way back until her head and arms are touching the floor (with pillows underneath). From here, the man will hold onto her hips and can move her body onto his penis at whatever speed and depth he wishes. He can also grab onto her breasts and massage her clitoris in this position if he wishes.

The Sitting Duck

Another position requiring complete trust is the sitting duck. This is a position that allows the woman to have complete control. The man will lie down on the floor on his back. The woman will straddle him and slide his penis into her. Then, one by one, she will cross her legs so that she is essentially sitting on his penis cross-legged. In this position, the man has no freedom of movement, and everything is up to the woman. She can even touch her clitoris in this position if she wishes.

Chapter 7: Advanced Kama Sutra Sex Positions

In this chapter, we are going to continue our examination of the Kama Sutra sex positions by looking at some of the more advanced positions. These positions will require more flexibility and strength from either the man, the woman or both.

While they require more strength and flexibility, they come with great rewards in the form of pleasure if you can get into them.

Advanced Kama Sutra Sex Positions

After reading through this list of advanced Kama Sutra sex positions, try some for yourself with your partner. Challenging yourselves to get into new sex positions will be an intimate and sexy experience that will benefit your relationship.

The Turning Position

The Turning Position is a fun one that you have probably never heard of before. It can add some fun into your stale sex life or some pizazz into a new and youthful relationship. This is one of the more challenging positions to master and requires quite a lot of communication from both parties. It will also require some practice to execute it seamlessly, but don't be intimidated; you will master it in no time and begin to wow all of your present and/or future partners! This position is well suited to couples who would like to try something different and explore new ways of reaching pleasure together at a point in their relationship when they are comfortable with each other and know how to communicate well.

The position begins in the classic Missionary position (as discussed previously in this book) with the man on top of the woman and both of them face to face. The man's legs should both be between the woman's legs, and his penis is already inside of her. This is where it gets more complicated, so listen closely. The man now lifts his left leg over the woman's right leg and then proceeds to lift his right leg over her right leg, keeping his penis inside of her, and continues by moving his upper body in a clockwise direction until he is at a 90-degree angle to her body, essentially lying across her (while still penetrating her). He will then move his legs over her upper body, one leg at a time, continuing to turn around in a clockwise direction so that his feet are at either side of her head, still maintaining the positioning of his penis inside her vagina. From here, he will complete the turn and come back to his starting Missionary position without ever removing his penis from her vagina. Doing this seamlessly and sensually without accidentally pulling out of her will require some practice and cooperation on both of their parts. When it is done well, it looks like he is turning in a slow and smooth circle around her body.

This position will lead to new sensations for both people as every single angle of his penis inside her vagina will be felt by both of them. It will lead to new challenges for both of them as it is a complex position to try. And it will lead to the exploration of new points of view of the other person's body, all three of these things leading to greater intimacy and closeness between partners.

The Scissors Position

This position is a little difficult to get yourselves into, but once you do, it will be well worth the effort. To begin, the man will sit on the bed with his arms behind him, holding his weight up but leaning back. Then, he will bend one of his knees, so his leg is bent. The woman will lie down on the bed face-down and with her head at the opposite end of the bed as the man. She will spread her legs and move her body toward the man's until their bodies meet. When they meet, their bodies will look like two pairs of scissors crossed into one another. From here, the man will insert his penis into her vagina. The woman can move her body up and down on his penis, and the man can thrust into her. It may take a bit of time to develop a rhythm in this position, but when you do, you will both feel intense pleasure.

The Plow

As the name suggests, this position is designed to make you emulate a human plow, but I assure you, this position is much sexier than it sounds. This position is a great introduction to some of the more interesting and difficult Kama Sutra sex positions. This is a great option if you wish to get acquainted with the world of Kamasutra for the first time and wish to challenge yourselves.

You, as the woman, lie face-down on the bed with your hips and legs sticking off the end and support yourself on your elbows. Your man stands on the floor beside the bed, his body positioned between your legs. He then lifts your lower half up by your hips and thighs and inserts his penis into your vagina, while supporting your legs the entire time. You can take a more passive role in this position, and he can adjust the angle he holds your legs at for maximum pleasure.

The Peg Position

The Peg has a sexy name that implies pleasure and may even have you turned on already. This is a more difficult position, certainly more difficult to get yourselves into, but it comes with the reward of a great all-encompassing orgasm for both parties if it can be done.

The man lies on his side, and the woman lies facing him on her side, with her head towards his feet. The woman will lift her knees towards her chest and place one of her legs underneath the man's legs and have the other on top of his legs. Essentially, she is hugging his legs with her entire body. She slides up so that her vulva is next to his penis. When aligned properly, he can penetrate her and can achieve depth and control as she is positioned perfectly for his penis to enter her. The woman wraps her arms around his legs, and he can use his hands and arms to help with his thrusting, or if she is comfortable, he can use his hands to stimulate her anal area with his fingers or a toy. The woman is positioned like this allows for all of her vulvae to be open and accessible once again, and this is what will lead to a stronger orgasm for her. The man being able to see all of her and to play with her anus will lead to a stronger orgasm for him.

The Posture of Splitting Bamboo

The woman will lie on her back and have the man lie on top of her, sliding his body in between her legs. The woman will lift one of her legs and put it on one of his shoulders, and the other will stretch out past his body. From here, he pushes his hips forward and can easily slide his penis into her vagina, which is open and in a perfect position for penetration. The man will do the thrusting here. After some time, the woman will switch and put the other leg on his other shoulder. She can continue to alternate as they engage in intercourse.

This position requires flexibility in the woman but gives a deep penetration once accomplished and almost rides that line between pleasure and pain due to the stretch.

This position allows for deep penetration as well as varied pressure on the man's penis, which will be extremely pleasurable for him.

If the woman is feeling flexible and wants to try a new position that will have both of them benefitting from a deeper penetration than most of the classics, this position will be a great choice.

The Suspended Congress

To get into this position, the man will stand facing a wall with the woman standing in front of him, her back to the wall. She will then jump into his arms and wrap both her arms and her legs around him. Once here, he can insert his penis into her vagina while holding onto her buttocks or underneath her knees. He can lean her back on the wall in front of him for support so that he does not have to support her entire weight in his arms. If he holds onto her underneath her knees, this will open her up so that her vagina is easily accessible. The fact that she is suspended coupled with this will make it so that there is deep penetration occurring, and this will be pleasurable for both the man and the woman. Deep penetration is great for the female orgasm because there are two places located deep within the vagina that, when stimulated, lead to a very intense orgasm for her. The penis must achieve continuous deep penetration in order for this to happen, and in this position, it is quite possible.

This position is great for the female orgasm because of the angle that the man's penis enters her vagina. It is also quite pleasurable for the woman because the man is in control in this position, so the woman can relax and enjoy the pleasure he is bringing to her body.

Crossed Keys

The Crossed Keys is a relatively simple position but makes for an interesting and new position to try if you have never done it before. This is a great introduction to the world of more complex and acrobatic positions. While this is not quite acrobatic, it will introduce you to this type of sex.

Have your woman lie down on her back at the edge of the bed with her legs sticking straight up into the air, knees straight. She then crosses one leg in front of the other, keeping them sticking straight up. Stand at the edge of the bed and grab a hold of her outstretched legs. Then, with your feet planted on the floor, slide your penis into her vagina and holding her legs as a stable base, you can thrust harder and faster as she likes it. With her legs crossed over each other like this, it tightens her vagina so that it creates a tighter and more pleasurable environment for your penis as well as creating more pleasure for her because the tighter vagina canal will mean more contact of your penis with the walls of her vagina and will lead to G-spot stimulation.

The Toad Position

This position is similar to The Toad (or The Frog) stretch that you may have done in a yoga class before. Facing the floor with bent knees spread wide to get those hips stretched. I bet you never thought that would help you in your sex life... But low and behold, turn that stretch over, and you have The Toad position! I will explain in more detail as follows.

The woman lays on her back, bending her knees towards her chest and spreading her knees open wide. This opens her body up for easy penetration, clitoris access, and maximum exposure of all of her pleasurable parts to her man's body that will be rubbing against them. The woman's entire vulva can be a pleasurable area if it is exposed to touch like the man's pelvis or hips rubbing it. This, coupled with the clitoris being rubbed at the same time, will drive her crazy. The man lies on top of her and slides his penis into her vagina, having lots of space for deep penetration. In this position, the woman's clitoris can easily be stimulated from the thrusting motion of the man's body on top of hers or from the base of his penis when he comes as close to her as possible with each thrust. If the woman wants to take more control, once he is inside of her, she can wrap her legs around his waist and use them to pull his hips towards her along with his movement to increase the pressure and depth of his penetration.

The Widely Opened Position

The name of this position means that the woman's entire body is widely opened to receive pleasure in the form of her man. Her body is in a position that says she is ready for this experience.

As the woman, lie down on a bed on your back with your man on top of you, both of his legs between yours. Have him hold his weight up, so he is hovering over you, allowing you to get into position before he comes into you. Proceed to throw your head all the way back so you can see your headboard and arch your back at the same time, pushing your breasts into the air. Use your elbows behind you to support you and lift your hips into the air to meet your man's body that is hovering over top of you. Hold onto this position and (in whatever sensual language you feel turned on by) invite your man to put his penis into you. While you hold yourself up in this position, he can then thrust his penis in and out with varying speed and force. If it proves to be too difficult for you to hold up your body weight the entire time, ask your man to help you by holding himself up with one arm, and by wrapping his other arm under your lower back to support you a bit.

So why hold your body in this difficult position you ask? The reason for this is that the woman's raised position allows the man to achieve deep penetration like the vagina is raised up and more exposed to the front where the man's penis is. Further, because she is pressed up in an arched-back position, her clitoris is lifted and exposed more than ever, which will allow for the friction of the man's thrusts against her body to stimulate the clitoris with each pump.

The Standing Position

The standing position may be a little difficult, but with practice, you might just add this one into your regular rotation. Many variations can be done with this position, depending on what feels best for both of you and how your stamina is.

To start, it may be easier to have the man standing against a wall so that he can lean his back onto it for support. The woman then will stand in front of the man, facing away from him. Now for the tricky part, you will need to play around a bit to find the right way for both of you to reach this. The man will now need to insert his penis into his female partner's vagina from behind. This will work best if the man leans back against the wall, lowering his body so that he can push his hips upward toward his partner's vulva. The woman can reach back and hold onto the man if she wishes.

The Fixing of a Nail

This is another position that involves the man on top of the woman in a position similar to the Missionary Position, but this is a more difficult variation.

In this position, the woman will place one of her legs on the man's head, and the other will be stretched out below her. The Kama Sutra states that this position will require a lot of practice to accomplish. Once you are able to do this position, you will benefit from a very deep penetration, as well as a high likelihood of G-Spot stimulation for the woman.

The Pressed Position

This position is a little challenging, but it has great benefits for those who can achieve it. This position requires a little bit of flexibility, but it also acts as a stretch, so if you ease into it you should be able to reach the full position within a few minutes after your body is warmed up.

To get into this position, the woman lies on her back and brings her knees to her chest, wrapping her arms around them, her body forming a small ball shape. The man kneels near her buttocks and enters her vagina from a kneeling position in front of her. Her vagina will be quite easily accessible because her legs are lifted at her chest. If the flexibility is there, the man can now lean forward with his upper body, and with his own chest, he can hold her legs to her chest for her so that her hands are free. With her free hands, she can hold the back of his neck, pull his hair, or caress his face, depending on what direction you want to go with this sexual encounter. From here, the man's penis can very easily meet the woman's G-spot because of its curve, and this will make for an intense orgasm for both parties. The restriction of movement paired with the extreme closeness of their bodies is sure to make for some pent-up arousal that has no other way to be released than through a full-body orgasm.

The Sphinx Position

The Sphinx gets its name from the ancient Egyptian sculptures of women in this type of position, although without the man penetrating her. These sculptures and statues were not erotic! But you can make your own erotic Sphinx at home after you read on about this position.

The woman lies face down, supporting herself on her elbows. She stretches one leg out behind her and bends the other out to the side of her body to spread out and open up access to her vagina. The man lies on top of the woman, and his penis enters her vagina from behind. This may be hard if he has a smaller penis, but he will need to get as low as possible, and it should still work! The weight of the man lying on top of the woman makes for added pleasure for her because it spreads her legs further apart so that her pleasure centers are more accessible. It also increases pressure on her pelvis, which will help in leading to an orgasm, and when it does, an even stronger and better orgasm because the pressure from the outside meets the pressure from the inside and voilà! Full body bliss.

X-Rated

The X-Rated is a position that the man will love if he has not already suggested it sometime in your relationship! You can probably glean this from the name though.

If you are the man, lie down on your back, and the woman will lie on top of you, facing down your body with her head at your feet. She will wrap her arms around your legs and spread her legs so that they are on either side of your hips. She can then slide up or down your body to adjust for ease of inserting your penis into her. If it is easier, start in reverse cowgirl (like we examined earlier in this book) and have her lie forward after you penetrate her so that she is lying on your legs. She can wrap her arms around your legs after this. Either you can pump your hips into her with her lying on your penis, or she can lift her hips up and down on your penis for the magic to happen. She can be in control of the depth and speed of penetration by doing this if you wish. You as the man in this position, will likely want your head propped up by a pillow or three so that you can take in the full view of your woman below the waist with her naked bum in the air, gyrating on your erection in all her beauty.

This position is loved by many men, but also by many women for the same reasons that they love reverse cowgirl. Deep penetration, the ability to be in control of the humping and G-spot stimulation. The trifecta of female pleasure!

Chapter 8: Other Kama Sutra Techniques

Now that you have gained a solid understanding of the sex positions that are included within the Kama Sutra, we are going to look at some of the other topics that the text discusses.

Techniques That Do Not Involve Penetration

As I mentioned in the first chapter of this book, the Kama Sutra contains much more than a list of sex positions. In this section, we are going to look at some of the other demonstrations of love that the Kama Sutra teaches.

These techniques are said to be intended for foreplay. They will help you and your partner to get in the mood by touching and kissing each other. They can also be done anytime that you wish to share some intimate moments with your significant other.

Kissing

The Kama Sutra discusses kissing as one of the many ways to connect with your partner, aside from having sexual intercourse. The Kama Sutra mentions kissing as a way to connect with your partner before sex, during sex, or any other time you wish.

There are numerous places that the Kama Sutra deems the "places for kissing." They are as follows;

- Forehead
- Cheeks
- Eyes
- Throat
- Bosom
- Breasts
- Lips
- Interior of the Mouth
- Joints of the Thighs
- Arms
- The navel

There are also different techniques for kissing. They are listed below.

1. The Normal/Nominal Kiss

A young girl kisses her partner with a small peck on the lips.

2. The Straight Kiss

When two people make contact with their lips.

3. The Turned Kiss

One partner holds the head and chin of the other partner and kisses them.

4. The Throbbing Kiss

When a young girl kisses her partner and moves only her bottom lip.

5. The Touching Kiss

The man and woman touch each other's hands, close their eyes, and the girl touches her partner's lips with her tongue.

6. The Bent Kiss

When the two kissers bend their heads and kiss.

7. The Pressed Kiss

When one partner kisses the lower lip of the other partner with force.

8. The Greatly Pressed Kiss

When one partner takes the lower lip of the other between two fingers and then touches the lip with their tongue using great force.

9. Kiss of the Upper Lip

When a man kisses the woman's upper lip, and she kisses his lower lip.

10. A Clasping Kiss

When one person takes both of the other person's lips with their lips. It is stated that a woman should only have this kind of kiss with a man who has no mustache.

11. The Kiss that Kindles Love

A woman looks at her partner's face while he is asleep and kisses it.

12. The Kiss That Turns Away

When a woman kisses a man while he is fighting with her, or while he is busy with business. This kiss happens when his mind is "turned away."

13. The Kiss That Awakens

When a man comes home late, and his wife is already asleep, he kisses her.

14. Kiss Showing The Intention

When a person kisses the reflection of their lover in a mirror or water.

15. The Transferred Kiss

When a person kisses a child, who is sitting on his lap or a picture while his lover is in the room.

16. The Demonstrative Kiss

When a man kisses a woman's finger if she is standing up, her toe if she is sitting down or while a woman is shampooing her lover's body.

Scratching and Biting

The following list includes several forms of biting which are done to show your partner that you love them. It can also be done as a type of foreplay if this person is turned on by biting.

- Swollen Bite
- Hidden Bite
- Point
- Line of Point
- Coral and the Jewel
- Line of the Jewels
- Broken Cloud
- Biting of the Boar

Striking

The Kama Sutra also talks about something called striking. This may come as a surprise to you, but striking is something that many people find pleasure in. Striking is a form of rough sex, but one that does not involve anything too serious in terms of the acts that it calls for.

Striking can be done in a gentle way, or in a firmer way, depending on what the couple themselves prefer. This can be seen as an introduction to rough sex. In today's world, rough sex is also sometimes referred to as BDSM. BDSM stands for Bondage, Discipline, Dominant and Submissive, Sadism, and Masochism. The four letters in this acronym overlap to mean a wide variety of things. Under this umbrella, there is something for everyone and probably many things that you didn't even know about that turn you on. It is all about finding pleasure without restrictions or judgment and letting yourself explore a different world of sex.

When comparing the striking techniques of the Kama Sutra to modern-day BDSM, many similarities can be drawn. More specifically, this technique could be compared to S&M. Sadism and masochism, commonly known as S&M, is the addition of pain play into your sexual experiences. The thin line between pleasure and pain is ridden here to give extreme pleasure mixed with a little bit of fear. The sadist is the person who gets pleasure from inflicting pain on their partner or rather is turned on by the power it has. The masochist is the person who gets pleasure from being in pain at the hands of their partner and riding the line between pleasure and pain.

Places You Can Strike

When it comes to striking, the Kama Sutra mentions six places that you can strike. They include the following;

- Head
- Shoulders
- Back
- Sides
- Between the breast
- The Jaghana (the buttocks)

The Ways You Can Strike

There are also 4 specific ways that you can strike. They include the following;

- Back of the Hand
- Fingers spread out
- With Open Hand
- With Fist

A Note on Sexual Compatibility

Concerning the techniques above that involves scratching, biting, and striking, one topic that this brings up is sexual compatibility. Firstly, what is Sexual Compatibility?

Sexual compatibility between people means that they share the same beliefs, values, preferences, desires, and expectations related to sex. This can include things like what sex acts you prefer the most, your level of sex drive, the type of sex you wish to have, including any fetishes, and so on. For example, if you have a very high sex drive, meaning that you need and expect to have sex every single day, you will be sexually compatible with someone who also has a high sex drive. If you were in a sexual relationship with someone who had a very low sex drive, this would be incompatible as you would likely become frustrated by their low need for frequent sex. Another example is if you desire a lot of oral sex and you require this in order to become fully aroused during sex, you would be sexually compatible with someone who also enjoys oral sex, especially giving it. If you were with someone who did not feel comfortable with oral sex at all, this would not make for a sexually compatible match.

Your preferences and values do not have to be exactly the same as the person you are in a sexual relationship with, but they must be able to fit together (like yin and yang) for a sexual relationship to be compatible. An example of this is if you enjoy slow and tender sex, but your partner enjoys rough sex. This could mean that you are sexually incompatible, but it could also work if you are both able to meet in the middle. You could start off by having slow and tender foreplay while your arousal builds, and when you are both ready for penetration, the sex can begin to lead towards a rougher style. As long as both people are comfortable with this, this sexual relationship could work.

When it comes to kinks and fetishes, sexual compatibility is quite important. For example, BDSM, including dominance and submission. If you have one partner who is sexually dominant and the other who prefers submission, this works out very well. If, however, you prefer dominance and so does your partner or if both prefer submission, you may have some trouble reaching a place of agreement when it comes to your sexual encounters. The dominant person will not usually become turned on by being told what to do, and the submissive person will usually not be too excited by telling someone else what to do. While these can work on a spectrum and people can enjoy a bit of both, many people are either dominant or submissive.

Taking this into account is important because when trying new things in the bedroom, it is important to ensure that you and your partner are both comfortable with the new techniques that you are introducing.

Double Oral Sex Technique: The Roll

This position is a wonderful oral sex position. Remember, as I mentioned that the book of Kama Sutra includes a variety of oral sex positions, not only positions in which to have intercourse. This is one of those positions.

In this position, the man will be stimulating the woman's anus and/or vagina orally while she gives him oral sex at the same time. To get into this position, the woman will lie on the bed on her back, and she will hold onto her ankles, spreading her legs out to the side as much as possible. The man will come over the woman, facing her feet, and he will place one of his knees on either side of her head, and one of his hands on either side of her hips. He will then lower himself down so that he can stimulate her orally. The woman will pull her ankles toward her head so that her body rolls up into a ball, giving the man more ease of access. She will then take his penis in her mouth and stimulate him orally. This position allows both people to benefit from oral sex at the same time. The man can also use one of his hands to stimulate the woman anally, vaginally, or clitorally while he gives her oral.

Oral Sex for Men

This position is done when the man is standing up, and the woman is on her knees in front of him, giving him oral sex. You may be thinking that this is not an advanced sex position because you have done it many times, and it is quite common. Here, however, we are going to make it an advanced position.

To make this into an advanced sex position, while the woman is kneeling in front of the man and giving him oral sex, she can use one of her hands to hold onto his testicles and gently massage them. This will add to his pleasure quite a bit. She can also (or instead) use her other hand to reach around behind him and stimulate his anus with her finger. She can move her finger around the outside of his anus, stimulating the sensitive skin there, and this will make him feel immense amounts of pleasure. Doing both of these at the same time will make it virtually impossible for him not to orgasm very quickly.

Oral Sex for Women

Similar to the previous position, this one may seem as if it is common and has been done a million times, however, with this position as well, we will be adding some elements that take it from an easier position to an advanced one.

To get into this position, the woman lies down on her back, and the man will lie down as well, but instead of lying down parallel to her with his mouth at her clitoris, he will lie down with his mouth at her clitoris but his body perpendicular to her. This way, their bodies form the letter 'T.' Lying like this makes it so that the woman can have the most pleasure possible from oral sex because it makes it easier for the man to stimulate her clitoris for a longer period without becoming fatigued. It is easier to move your tongue in an up and down motion than in a side to side motion, and when forming a T with their bodies, his tongue can move up and down (side to side on the clitoris) and give her the most pleasure possible. This is because stimulating the clitoris in this way is the most likely to lead to orgasm, whereas moving over it in a top to bottom motion will not lead to as much pleasure or as much chance of orgasm. When lying in a classic oral sex position of the man between the woman's legs, it would be hard for him to move his tongue in a side to side motion for a long time as it would become very fatigued, but if he moves his tongue up and down, it will not be as pleasurable for her. For these reasons, this T position is the best choice for oral sex for a woman.

Chapter 9: The Kama Sutra Theories of Romance

In this chapter, we are going to look at the Kama Sutra in terms of the way it discusses romance. There are a variety of tips that the Kama Sutra contains, which are related to romance, including tips for cuddling and embracing. We will then look at some Kama Sutra theories of relationships. The Kama Sutra outlines various relationships that we will look at in this chapter.

Kama Sutra Cuddling and Embracing

The first embrace we will discuss is called *The Milk and Water Embrace.* This position gets its name from the idea that the two people in this position are enmeshed and become so close that they lose themselves in the other person. Interestingly, this position can be used as a loving embrace after sex or a cuddle before sex.

The man sits on the edge of the bed, his legs planted on the floor. The woman approaches him and climbs into his lap, her face to his. She wraps her legs around his waist and her arms around his neck. He holds onto her by wrapping his arms around her back. The woman is pressed against her man, and this is a great position for cuddling, or she can keep both arms around his neck for a closer embrace.

This position is quite easy to get into and only requires a bit of strength from the man. Both of their bodies are supporting each other in this position, which is what makes it so intimate. Their bodies are touching at every point from head to toe, and they can breathe together and feel each other's heartbeat. This is why this position is said to be two people becoming one, like mixing milk and water when you can't tell where one ends, and the other begins.

From here, if they wish to transition in this position to penetrative sex, the woman can position herself so that her legs are open wide and receive his penis. To begin thrusting, they can work together, with the man using his feet on the floor as support. He can move his hips up and down, and the woman can grind her hips on his lap for pleasurable clit stimulation. If she wants, the woman can touch herself during this movement for extra pleasure.

The Kama Sutra also mentions several positions for cuddling and embracing aside from the Milk and Water Embrace. These other positions can be included after sex or during a time when you and your partner wish to hold each other and share an intimate moment.

Each time you make love with your partner, it is a bonding experience resulting in increased closeness. Each of these experiences of lovemaking contributes to your shared moments and your intimacy. Because of this, post-sex behavior is very important.

After a great orgasm, you probably collapse on top of each other, short of breath and muscles tired. Having made love, you are probably feeling quite close and romantic with each other since you have made each other feel warm and pleasured like no other. Therefore, after collapsing into each other, you will likely want to be as close as possible. We are going to look at some of the closest and romantic positions for that after-sex recovery cuddle.

First is the *head on chest* cuddle. Lie down on your back with your partner lying beside you on their side, their head resting on your chest or in the crook of your neck. In this position, you can hold each other with your arms wrapped around their body, and you can give your partner soft forehead kisses.

Second is the spooning position. Both of you will lie on your sides facing the same direction, with your bodies pressed against each other. Spooning is a position in which you can have sex as well, with the man behind the woman. This position is good for a lazy Sunday morning when you are both sleepily horny for each other. If you have just finished having sex in this position, you can nicely transition to cuddling in this same position right after he pulls out of her. When he finishes, he can then wrap his arms around her and kiss her softly on the cheek.

These cuddling positions are perfect for the after-sex whispered conversation that often happens when you have sex in a relationship. You can tell the person that what they just did to you made you feel amazing, or that they were so sexy when they did that certain thing. You can share words like "*I love you"* and gentle kisses.

If you want a position that allows you to share kisses on the lips and gazes into each other's eyes, this next position will be best for you. Lie on your sides facing each other with your legs intertwined and your faces just inches from each other. From here, you can romantically gaze into their soul and enjoy the after-sex glow on your partner's face.

A common practice after sex is that you may also want to share the intimacy of a nap together. Any of these cuddling positions previously mentioned will be perfect for a post-sex nap. The tiredness that you feel after an orgasm is best accompanied by a cat nap with your lover. The vulnerability of sleeping naked together is something you don't share with just anyone and is a special moment with the person you love.

We are all busy people in this day and age, and sometimes we won't have time to lie around with our partner after sex. So how do we maintain that intimacy of a post-sex cuddle if we have just squeezed in a quickie before breakfast and the kids will wake up soon? The deeper idea here is the connection and making time for our partner. Spending time after sex is a way of showing each other that despite the busy lives we lead, we are still doing life together and share a bond with them that we don't share with anyone else. There are other ways to show this post-sex if you simply don't have time for a cuddle. However, I would encourage you to try to set aside even two to three minutes after sex to get into a close embrace with your partner and to just enjoy their presence without the distraction of life or even of the act of sex. To come together without any sort of action and get quiet together.

Kama Sutra Theories of Relationships

There are a variety of different relationships that are discussed in the Kama Sutra. Some of these relationships are between a woman and a man who are married, some are between a man and his mistress, and others involve group relationships. Below I have outlined some of the different relationships that the Kama Sutra talks about, including how the Kama Sutra says that these individuals should interact when it comes to sex.

Before moving on, note that Kama Sutra discusses sex using the term *Congress*. You will see examples of this below.

The United Congress

The United Congress refers to a sexual encounter involving one man and two women. The Kama Sutra mentions that a man should enjoy sex with two women at the same time, both of whom love him equally.

When a man is having sex with two women at once, this is called the *United Congress*.

The Congress of the Herd of Cows

The Kama Sutra also mentions group sex, though it may not be the type of group sex that you would expect. The type of group sex that is discussed in the text involves many women and one single man.

When a man is enjoying sex with many women, this called *Congress of the Herd of Cows*.

The Gramaneri

Another form of group sex that is discussed in the Kama Sutra is something called *The Gramaneri*.

This kind of group sex involves many men that are having sex with one woman. The woman involved is usually married to one of the men who are present in this group sexual encounter. In this scenario, there are two options. The men could opt to have sex with the woman one at a time, each of the men taking a turn.

Alternatively, all of the men could have sex with the woman at the same time. For this option, the Kama Sutra specifies the following arrangement; One man holds the woman, another man penetrates her vaginally, another man is given oral sex by her, and another holds her "middle part." Then, they will alternate and continue to "enjoy her" in all areas, taking turns at each part of her body.

Keep in mind that the Kama Sutra was written long ago. It was written to be read by men. Further, it was written in a time and place where a man could have multiple women at the same time, even if he was married.

Conclusion

The hope is that this book has given you the tools you need to keep your sex life fresh and ever-changing by introducing you to the world of Kama Sutra. Maybe you have tried some of the positions from the Kama Sutra before, and you needed help to learn more. Maybe you are new to sex, and you wanted to study up on different positions to try for beginners. You now have a whole arsenal of positions to try. Maybe you have tried all of the classics and are looking to get into something completely new and adventurous. Whatever experience you came with, I hope that you are leaving this book having learned a few new things to take with you into your sexual adventures from here forward. I hope this serves as a tool for you to explore and discover yourself and your future partners.

What to Do Next?

As you go on in your sexual life, stay open-minded, and never stop listening to your body. People change, and you will likely change as well. By being open to these changes and being receptive to them in yourself and your long-term partner, you will be able to ensure you are always getting the most out of sex. Don't forget to communicate with your partner to better understand them and sex in general, all communication leads to learning, and this is a great thing when it comes to sex and relationships.

There is something for everyone in this book, so continue to pass it on to your friends and your partners so that we can live in a world of educated and informed sexual beings. The Kama Sutra is a guidebook for love and everything involved in loving another person. It is more than just a book of sex positions, but these days most people only know it for its complex and flexibility-requiring positions for intercourse. The book of Kamasutra includes a general guide to living well in ways other than through sex. It includes a guide to foreplay, a guide to kissing and touching, as well as other ways to achieve intimacy with your partner, such as bathing together and giving each other massages. I hope that after reading this book, you understand and can appreciate this text in a new way.

In addition to the positions enclosed in these pages, I hope that you learned how to focus on your pleasure and the pleasure of your partner, how to be present during sex, and how to become more sexually intuitive, to feel the most pleasure possible. What a waste of pleasure it would be to always have sex in the same positions over and over and never fully reach your potential for orgasm! If you haven't already, try some of the things you've learned through reading this book, and I assure you that your sex life will be much better for it!

You are now ready to go off into the world of sexual exploration and have great orgasms from here on out. Stay curious and keep learning!

How to Benefit from the Kama Sutra for Life

1. New Sex Positions

After reading about the sex positions of the Kama Sutra, you can now incorporate them into your own sex life. Read back through the chapters on sex positions with your partner and try these new positions with them. This will make for a fun and interesting experience for the two of you. Who knows, you may even find a new favorite position for intercourse.

2. New Relationship Dynamics

As I mentioned previously, though it is an ancient book, the Kama Sutra mentions same-sex relations. Within the book, same-sex relations are referred to as *the third nature*. As I mentioned, it also talks about group sex and group relationships. What this means is that although the Kama Sutra was written so long ago, in some ways, it has become more and more relevant over the years. As our modern-day relationships have shifted and changed, the Kama Sutra has stood the test of time. In some ways, it can be said that this book has aged well.

3. New Fantasies and Kinks to Explore

In addition to talking about group sex and same-sex encounters, the Kama Sutra also recognizes that there are many different ways that people find sexual satisfaction. The Kama Sutra allows for the exploration of a person's *kinks*. For example, the Kama Sutra mentions rough sex and how it can bring sexual pleasure and satisfaction to some. As kinks and fetishes have become more widely accepted in our world, this book has begun to show that it has aged well in yet another way.

This book is here to provide you with everything you want to know about the Kama Sutra and so much more! Do yourself a favor, your partner a favor, and everyone that you will ever have sex with favor by reading this book and teaching yourself as much as you possibly can. Give your partner the gift of informing yourself about how to please them like never before using these ancient but ever-relevant positions. All you have to do is click that download button, and you will be able to begin your journey to becoming the best sexual being you have ever been!

Description

This book will teach you everything you have ever wondered about the Kama Sutra!

Firstly, what is Kama Sutra? When we say the term *Kama Sutra*, it is actually about an ancient book. You may not have been aware of this fact, as most of the time we talk about Kama Sutra as a type of sex. While this book does guide you through sex by teaching you sex positions, it is a guide rather than a style of sex.

You will learn details like this and much more inside of this book.

This book will teach you;

- What the Kama Sutra is
- What the different sections of the Kama Sutra contain
- The benefits of the Kama Sutra
- How the Kama Sutra can improve your sex life
- How to better connect to your partner on more than a physical level for more passionate lovemaking
- Specific positions from The Kama Sutra to use in any situation you could imagine!
- How to develop intimacy and use this to have the best sex of your life!
- How to give better oral sex with the secrets to male and female oral sex pleasure

- How to perform various Kama Sutra sex positions
- Kama Sutra techniques for kissing, biting, embracing, etc.

The Kama Sutra provides you with a multitude of ways to keep your relationship and your sex life interesting. In a long-term relationship, you may feel that you are becoming bored or that your sex life is becoming stale. By reading through the Kama Sutra in its entirety, you can discover ways to keep not only your sex life but your relationship interesting. Maybe you will find a new way to massage or cuddle that you hadn't considered before. Maybe you will find a new technique for oral sex that your partner will love. There are techniques like this for improving your relationship as a whole by keeping it new and interesting.

This book contains everything and anything you want and need to know about taking your exploration of sex to the next level through an understanding of Kama Sutra and its many benefits. Using the techniques and knowledge contained within these pages, The Kama Sutra, in combination with an exploration of Sex Toys, Sexual Fantasies, and role play, will help you impress your sexual partner. You will learn things you didn't even know you needed to know, but that will make you wonder how you ever lived without them!

This book is here to provide you with everything you want to know about the Kama Sutra and so much more! Do yourself a favor, your partner a favor, and everyone that you will ever have sex with favor by reading this book and teaching yourself as much as you possibly can. Give your partner the gift of informing yourself about how to please them like never before using these ancient but ever-relevant positions. All you have to do is click that download button, and you will be able to begin your journey to becoming the best sexual being you have ever been!

www.ingramcontent.com/pod-product-compliance
Lightning Source LLC
Chambersburg PA
CBHW050734030426
42336CB00012B/1567